*TINNITUS*

*HUMAN HORIZONS SERIES*

# TINNITUS

*Living with Noises in Your Head*

## MICHAEL O'TOOLE

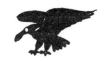

*A Condor Book*
*Souvenir Press (E&A) Ltd*

*In memory of my brother Gerard,
whose tinnitus was a greater burden
than anyone should bear*

First published 1995 by
Souvenir Press (Educational & Academic) Ltd,
43 Great Russell Street, London WC1B 3PA
and simultaneously in Canada

ISBN 0 285 63283 3

Typeset by Galleon Typesetting, Ipswich
Printed in Great Britain by
The Guernsey Press Co. Ltd, Guernsey, Channel Islands

# Contents

1 What is Tinnitus?   1
   Who has it?   5
   How people get tinnitus   10
   Tinnitus and young people   12

2 Looking for Relief   18
   Self-help   22
   In the mind   26
   Is it worse than total deafness?   28
   Family support   32

3 Mechanical Aids   38
   Gadgets for the home   38
   Hearing-aids   42
   Maskers   47

4 Professional Help   50
   Counselling   51
   Questions and answers   54

5 Alternative Therapies   68
   Hypnotism   68
   The Tomatis method   71
   Acupuncture   73
   Shiatsu   76
   Cranio-sacral massage   77
   Craniofacial therapy   79

6   Living with Tinnitus                         81
    Relaxation                                   82
    Avoiding the worst moments                   85
    Can diet make a difference?                  89
    Care of the ears                             91
    Hypersensitive ears                          94
    Sounds that are not there                    96
    Attitudes to tinnitus                        99
    Does flying affect tinnitus?                101
    The tinnitus alphabet                       104

7   Legal and Social Issues                     107
    Noise regulations in the workplace          107
    Claiming compensation                       110
    Tinnitus and incapacity benefit             112
    The invisible war wound                     114
    The NHS and tinnitus                        118
    A tinnitus manifesto                        122

8   The Search for a Cure                       128

9   Tinnitus and the Future                     135


The British Tinnitus Association                141

The Tinnitus Population of the UK               146

Useful Addresses                                147

Index                                           151

# 1   What is Tinnitus?

Ancient civilisations used to make holes in the head to get rid of the sound of evil spirits. Not much progress had been made by the sixteenth century, when a distracted woman wrote in her diary: 'My God, it is the Devil's noises.' And recently the London mother of a ten-year-old boy told their doctor: 'It is like a swarm of bees in his head, and he cries a lot.' Hundreds of millions of people throughout the world know what tinnitus is like, but still remain ignorant about precisely what it is.

It can be defined quite easily: sound inside the head not caused by anything outside it—the Latin word *tinnitus* literally means 'a ringing'. Quite unrelated to any external stimulus, it is confined to the head and cannot be heard by anyone else. To describe the sounds takes a little longer: they may resemble almost anything from a hissing to the roar of a jet engine. The commonest include metallic banging, whistling, drum beats, water running, electric drills, clock chimes and telephone bells. A single sound may be isolated or be joined intermittently or constantly by any of the others. The racket can be experienced in one or both ears or somewhere in the centre of the head. At its worst it can threaten mental health or lead a sufferer to suicide. Its prevalence and intensity make it one of the scourges of human life. It is also one of the most baffling.

Doctors are keen to point out that it is not a disease or malfunction of the body, but a symptom of something else. It is a medical condition. Once that is stated, further explanation becomes wafer thin. Attempts to add to the

basic knowledge of the subject become lost in the labyrinths
and byways of medical speculation and conjecture. If it is a
symptom, of what is it a symptom? When anything is said to
be symptomatic of something else, surely the 'something
else' cannot be a mystery? The symptom and the cause are
related and one cannot exist without the other. This line of
enquiry can bring about a shuffling of feet and a glazed
expression even among those who have studied the subject
professionally. Four thousand years ago the Egyptians had
something to say about rackety heads, but current theories
on what causes them still have to be proved. The status of
'symptom' must remain, but without compelling scientific
knowledge of the causes.

So what? a person plagued by tinnitus may reply. Isn't it
possible to cure it, symptom or not, without first proving
what started it, just as an aspirin helps a headache?

At present neither cure nor cause has been discovered or
defined. It can be relieved, and even seemingly abolished in
extremely rare cases as a result of protracted treatment, but
in statistical terms it remains an incurable condition.

Expectations that a single cure will be found are becoming increasingly unrealistic. Scientists now think there are
several causes and if this is the case, several cures will be
needed. The good news is that some forms of relief can be
applied to various forms of tinnitus whatever their causes
are. Treatment is therefore racing ahead of a cure or cures.

Because of its subjective and personal nature, tinnitus is a
challenge to good health which itself can be challenged by
sufferers, as later chapters of this book reveal. With determination and a positive outlook, it is possible to intervene successfully in the course of events when tinnitus strikes and discover
ways of getting the better of what at first can seem like a noisy
monster invading the head. Some simple therapies under the
direction of skilled people and, just as valuably, a few basic
pieces of advice can lighten the burden.

The new sufferer will be regaled with scores of highly
dubious 'remedies' deserving of the title quack medicine.

Practitioners of some of the more boastful branches of alternative medicine, who claim with scant evidence that they have the key to healthier living, have latterly added tinnitus to their lists. At the same time, there are treatments—on the fringe of conventional medicine—with credible testimonials from people with tinnitus, which warrant investigation.

Certainly it is not easy to make much progress in the partial defeat of tinnitus without accepting the psychological element in it. As it is a perceived noise, which others cannot hear, the processes of thought and sensations are heavily involved. It is therefore wrong to think of tinnitus as an ear-based affliction only, although the temptation to do so is great, as sounds and the hearing of them are fundamental to the ear. The outer ear, which is the part most of us see, and essentially collects the sounds being received, can be eliminated from investigations into the cause of tinnitus. The middle ear is a fairly simple section, carrying sounds to the drum. Modern surgery can clear blockages and repair damage there. The inner ear, with the cochlea, reveals a vastly complicated world, however, with nerve connections to the part of the brain dealing with hearing. Damage through injury or ageing can play havoc with these microcomplex auditory pathways and is strongly suspected of being a cause of tinnitus. It is even thought that when certain signals fail to travel correctly or at all, the brain interprets their absence as a signal in itself and perversely creates sounds from what should be silence. If physical malfunctions of the inner ear are suspected of causing tinnitus, they cannot be treated. Indeed, the medical world cannot offer much, compared with the triumphs of drugs and surgery in relieving or curing other conditions. This is usually a dismal discovery for the new sufferer, who may think that the wonders of science are bound to have some solution. Nor is there much to cheer him or her up when he learns of what is being done to relieve tinnitus and to find a cure. One in ten adults, and many children, suffer from it, but the combined

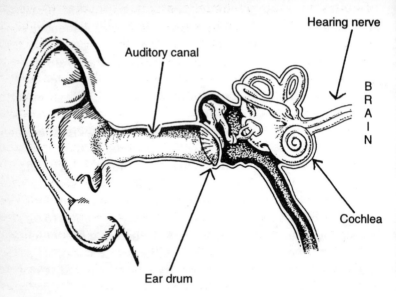

*External sound entering the ear travels along the auditory canal and causes the eardrum of the middle ear to vibrate. Through small bones the vibrations reach the inner ear and are changed into electrical impulses, which are received and interpreted by the brain as sound. It is thought that most tinnitus starts in the inner ear.*

*If the middle ear is found to be causing tinnitus, it is very occasionally possible to stop the sounds with surgery.*

resources of GPs' surgeries, hospitals and research establishments have, by truly scandalous neglect, pushed tinnitus way down the list of priorities.

Now, gradually, tinnitus is edging its way towards more sympathetic understanding in medicine and, slowly, among the policy-makers and politicians whose decisions can direct resources to the subject. Changes in priorities amid competing claims for other disabilities and afflictions will take time, however. Sufferers should not just wait for better treatment and a commitment to greater scientific research. The best advice is to act in the interim on their own behalf.

Tinnitus has many common consequences, some of which are likely to be suffered by anyone with all but the slightest sounds in the head. These can include insomnia and depression, both of which need a doctor's advice. It is a terrible mistake to conclude that because these conditions are caused by incurable tinnitus, they are also somehow beyond treatment. Nor should a reluctance to take drugs stand in the way. Similarly, the stress and anxiety which can follow from head sounds do not have to be tolerated. Once banished the tinnitus will appear to be reduced.

Worst of all, perhaps, is the overwhelming feeling of social isolation which new and chronic sufferers may encounter. The sounds can build a barrier between the person hearing them and the rest of society, especially if there is also serious deafness. This leads to introspection which strengthens the disinclination to reach out to non-sufferers. As the real cause is hidden, others do not understand. There are many paths to establishing a comfortable link with the rest of the world, and it would be naive to point to one for everyone to follow.

Many sufferers show inspiringly what can be achieved if, as Hamlet mused, they 'take arms against their sea of troubles'.


WHO HAS IT?

Second only to the shock of first encountering tinnitus in one's own head, the biggest surprise is finding out how many others have it. Look at a hundred people in a supermarket and about ten of them can be reckoned to have permanent sounds. Most will not be troubled, but one or two will be—even to the point of finding that the quality of their life is badly affected, maybe ruining their careers. In addition, research has shown, for every hundred people able to visit a supermarket, there will be one person so devastated that he cannot perform such an everyday task as shopping.

A thorough, nationwide survey conducted in the 1980s revealed that one in ten of the adult population has permanent tinnitus. That gives a formidable total of more than four million in the UK. A smaller percentage of teenagers and children are similarly affected (see table, p. 146).

A breakdown of statistics shows the real extent and seriousness of it all. Of every 100 men and women with tinnitus, 25 find it moderately annoying, for 15 it is severely annoying, ten find their quality of life badly affected and five say their normal, everyday life is severely affected. About 200 adults experience the onset of tinnitus every day, but rather more than half of all those who have the condition find it only slightly annoying or are not unduly troubled by it.

The problem is worldwide. Where reliable surveys have been conducted, the one in ten figure has been equalled, or exceeded. In the United States the total has reached an estimated 50 million. The less reliable evidence of anecdotal history and individual doctor's assessments also suggests that the British percentages are present across the world.

Up to now, very little effort has been made to quantify the economic and social cost of tinnitus in a whole population. Until this is done, governments remain to be persuaded that resources can legitimately be diverted to relieve or cure the condition, not knowing what net financial savings, if any, would follow from successful research and treatment. One telling piece of evidence has come from the former West Germany. It has been found that at least 5 million people over sixteen cannot follow the career of their choice because of their noises.

With a history, however sketchy, of thousands of years, tinnitus has many famous and infamous figures among its victims. In modern times Adolf Hitler was probably the best known. He kept it a close secret, confiding only in a doctor who later told all. It is not certain when the noises started, but they were made much worse by the explosion of the bomb when some of Hitler's officers tried to assassinate him in 1944. (One could speculate that the intense day and night distraction indirectly contributed to the desperate decisions taken in the Berlin bunker as the Allies closed in on the city.)

Artists of all kinds have left the world vivid and dramatic descriptions. The Spanish painter, Goya, found it to be a source of real anguish and Vincent van Gogh's self-mutilation in cutting off his ear is believed to be an extreme attempt to find relief.

Thomas Hardy used a character in *A Pair of Blue Eyes*, William Worm, to describe the affliction: 'I've got such a noise in my head . . . 'tis for all the world like people frying fish . . . sometimes 'tisn't only fish, but rashers of bacon and onions. Ay, I can hear the fat pop and fizz as natural as life.' The clergyman to whom he confided this was sympathetic enough, but confessed to being totally ignorant of the subject. Mr Worm showed some courage in his words, as people in those days were often labelled insane or mentally deficient and in need of some kind of custody if they complained of invisible rackets in the head. Jonathan Swift puzzled readers by writing of 'a thousand roaring oceans about my head' and in recent years Salman Rushdie, in his novel *Midnight's Children*, speaks of 'ringing bells of deafness'.

But it is musicians who have supplied the starkest descriptions for posterity. To find a reason for this, one has only to consider the effect loud and discordant sounds can have on people whose intellect is enveloped in the creation of melody and harmony.

The world knows Beethoven was deaf. A common image of him is sitting grumpily in a Viennese coffee house or at home in his ramshackle lodgings trying to converse with the assistance of an ear-trumpet.

It is virtually impossible to imagine what almost total deafness really meant to a genius writing music which changed mankind's view of life and the world. Think further and try to realise what terrible tinnitus meant to him.

For music lovers with tinnitus the house, now a small museum, in the Viennese suburb of Heiligenstadt where Beethoven wrote his famous Testament is a moving centre of pilgrimage. In 1802, at the age of thirty-two, he used the

document (actually a letter to his family) to describe his
shattering anguish and withdrawal from the social pleasures
of his youth.

> Though endowed with passionate and lively tempera-
> ment and even fond of the distractions offered by
> society, I was soon obliged to seclude myself and live
> in solitude. My misfortune pains me doubly, inasmuch
> as it leads to my being misjudged, for there can be no
> relaxation in human society, no refined conversations,
> no mutual confidences. I must live quite alone and may
> creep into society only as often as sheer necessity
> demands. At the age of 28 I was obliged to become a
> philosopher.

The Heiligenstadt Testament, written while Beethoven
was busy with the Second Symphony, stands today as a
monumental affirmation of the human spirit and its defiance
in the face of a medical condition scarcely more understood
today than it was in the early part of the nineteenth century.

Nor was there anything to be done for Robert Schumann,
whose deranged mental state was aggravated by tinnitus.
No one will ever know how much it contributed to his
unsettling illnesses, suicide attempts and early death.

In 1874, and at the height of his creative powers, the
Czech composer Smetana wrote to a colleague that a 'cruel
fate' had overtaken him. He told of 'buzzing and tingling in
my ears as if I were standing in a huge waterfall'. Before his
last days in a Prague lunatic asylum the composer revealed
his awful state of mind:

> That ringing in my head, that noise . . . is worst of all.
> Deafness would be a relatively tolerable condition if
> only all was quiet in my head. However, almost con-
> tinuous internal noises which sometimes increase to a
> thunderous crashing torture me greatly. This inex-
> plicable pandemonium is pierced by the shrieking of

voices, from strident whistles to ghastly bawling, as
though furies and demons were bearing down on me in
a violent rage . . . I begin to wonder what the end will
be . . .

In the twentieth century tinnitus has continued to take its
toll among both classical and pop musicians, with even
more concertgoers forced to give up their music. Some
performers, however, fight back successfully and overcome
their handicap sufficiently to continue their careers. In the
opera world one of the most successful recoveries has been
made by the singer Benjamin Luxon, who thought he
would have to retire when tinnitus replaced much of his
hearing. He now wears a hearing-aid as he treads the
opera stage and recital platform, and encourages others
too to fight back instead of despairing. Another type of
singer, Barbra Streisand, shares Mr Luxon's resolve, but
admits that strenuous public performances place an enormous strain on her, making her tinnitus much worse on
occasions.

Ronald Reagan, when United States president, found
his White House duties were made more taxing because
of his troublesome sounds. Many other statesmen and
politicians have deliberately kept quiet about what they
but no one else can hear, perhaps for fear of diminishing their purposeful standing among the electorate and
thereby being seen as not up to the task of leadership. By
and large they prefer not to talk about tinnitus, however
long they have had it. Two exceptions in the House of
Commons are the Liberal Democrat spokesman Robert
Maclennan and the Labour MP Don Dixon; the latter
blames a noisy ship-building yard, where he worked
before entering Parliament, for his trouble, which he
finds really bothers him after a long Commons debate. The
Speaker's time-honoured call of 'Order! Order!' is never
heeded inside his head.

# HOW PEOPLE GET TINNITUS

A constable was standing in the car-park at the police station where he worked when a roof slate fell on his head. At that moment he became one of the average of 200 people who experience the onset of tinnitus each day. The same fate awaited a youth when kicked in the neck in a rugby scrum. A thirty-year-old mother driving to school to collect her child was involved in a slight accident. She found that the whiplash effect caused by the collision brought with it a mixture of head sounds.

Most people, however, cannot point to a specific incident, but can usually say on what day—perhaps the hour and minute—it began. This exposes a paradox, that although tinnitus still insists on being an enigma wrapped in a mystery, it announces its attachment to an individual unequivocally and with a timing and precision lacking in most other medical conditions. This distinction would probably remain merely academic were it not for the fact that knowing when and in what circumstances it started can have a bearing on useful treatment. The policeman, for example, could have sustained a slight fracture of the skull, with the tinnitus serving some purpose in revealing the whole picture of the injury. The rugby player and the motorist could have sustained disruption of the neck or shoulder, and treatment for these injuries could well reduce the consequent tinnitus. Anyone new to tinnitus should try to recall any injury, however slight, before the noises commenced and mention the possible connection when seeing a doctor. But treatable physical injury associated with head noise accounts for only a small fraction of reported cases.

The trigger can be a surge of music at a pop concert, well above the decibel safety level, an explosion, a burst of gunfire, or surgery conducted on the ear or close to it. The list is a long one and has never been fully written. Even so it is of more anecdotal than scientific value to be able to pin-point the circumstances when the internal sounds began. It does not, for all its precise timing, help to reveal exactly what happened to the ears and the brain when excessive sounds lasting perhaps seconds left behind them other sounds for life. Did the sonic impact shake the nerves between the ears and the brain so badly that the hearing system was left incapable of accurately conducting messages for conscious, aural perception? Even to ask that is to speculate more than explain. At the same time, it does help some people to know of a link between, say, a blow or a loud bang and their tinnitus. It goes some way to rationalise the baffling business and to anchor their problem in a single explicable event that may have caused it, however mysteriously.

There is a list of things it is well to avoid, from discos and pop concerts to firing-ranges, if no ear protection is worn. One day, taking care of the ears and the dangers of exposing them to excessive noise will be included in health education.

There are many internal sounds without a causal link, however superficial. 'I woke up one day and it had just started' or 'I was sitting quietly reading a book when I heard what I thought were plumbing noises from the next room' are the sort of statements a family doctor hears in the surgery. They vastly out-number stories of kicks, accidents or big bangs. In a perverse way, it could be said that these totally unexplained beginnings of tinnitus correspond most accurately to the totally perplexing nature of the condition itself.

It is to some extent age related. A seventy-year-old stands a greater chance of getting it than a seventeen-year-old. There has been a tendency among some doctors to point to another mystery, the ageing process of the body, and say patients should accept tinnitus as easily and naturally as they accept growing old. When pressed to explain the spread of tinnitus through the age groups, they are tempted to round off their theory by saying that parts of the body can age prematurely. If it is possible for a man to be bald at thirty, why not tinnitus thirty or forty years earlier than one could reasonably expect it? The reasoning is rather thread-bare, and at best supplies only a part of the answer.

If a physical, external blow can disturb the ear-brain mechanism and bring on tinnitus, can a psychological condition start it in the brain, causing equal disturbance? Can the power of thoughts troubled by distress and anxiety, for instance, shatter internal silence just as external blows or sounds can, from the other direction?

The burden of personal worry, if not somehow released through the sharing of it with others, or diminished by a third party such as a skilled therapist, can bring about physical illness and malfunction of the metabolism. The mind dictates to an extent the course of health, and manifests its power in ways that illustrate persuasively the unique and abiding one-ness of mind and body. Research into tinnitus underlines the importance of the brain in the false and disruptive perception of sound that has no external source. It also seems that a mind plagued with anguish, probably unexpressed by the sufferer, is capable of originating the din that no one else can hear.


## TINNITUS AND YOUNG PEOPLE

A little boy of four once tugged at his father's arm and asked: 'Daddy, why does the brain make so much noise?' It was the first the puzzled parent knew that the infant was carrying around inside him a non-stop din that the majority of the population would never suffer. When tinnitus was diagnosed it was thought likely to have started at birth.

The boy became another one of the children and teenagers facing life with an incurable medical condition with the potential to hamper or even cripple career and social life. Although no statistical research on a national basis has yet been recorded, it is known that tinnitus is not as common among the young as it is in older people, and is therefore less than one person in ten. But for reasons special to the second half of the twentieth century, the situation is likely to get worse.

Loud noise or sound can cause tinnitus, and the sheer volume of much pop music is a culprit. Decibel levels at many rock concerts, which would be measured as illegal at places of work if ear protectors were not provided for employees, can either instantly damage those present or may do so years later; the effect waiting like a time bomb to explode. Identical dangers are inherent in domestic stereo equipment and personal Walkman-type headphones used wrongly; worst of all are discos, at which loud amplified sounds are made worse by the often sonic, confined nature of the location. Technology has, in the space of a few decades, brought massive sounds of an unprecedented nature within the reach of the general public. Science has outstripped the capacity of the human ear, and popular music, such a beguiling source of pleasure for millions, has left a vile visiting card. Social scientists point to the phenomenon of pop musical culture as both a harbinger and expression of youthful emancipation since the Second World War. The modern cult of the teenager has seen loud music become inseparable from the young's shout of defiance as adolescence cuts loose from convention. Any parent will agree it is hopeless to tell a son or daughter they should think of their ears as they go out to a disco or retreat to the bedroom with tapes and headphones. Still less will young people agree that they are stooges to a section of the ever-expanding music industry more interested in profits than in the health of their adoring customers.

GPs report a growing number of patients in school or college or in the early days of employment coming to their surgeries with ear problems. If they have tinnitus, it is now usual to ask if they have been exposed to loud music. Many patients say the noises started at a disco or concert or soon afterwards. More often than not they had expected any instant noise in the head to last just an hour or so. But the sounds—which, of course, bear no direct relation to what was heard from the stage—will still be present in the head when the memory of their favourite pop group has long faded.

The portable and easily afforded cassette player, complete with headphones, has become a universal symbol of youth, worn unselfconsciously on the bus, in the street, on bikes and in the park. Used recklessly, it is also a dangerous weapon. If a Walkman-type player can also be heard by another person six feet or more away, the wearer is risking tinnitus.

While it is only the sufferer who can describe it, and it cannot yet be measured scientifically, the step of sound at which tinnitus can be triggered is known. Disco music can reach 115 decibels or more. The danger threshold is 80 decibels and health campaigners claim that government health warnings, rather like those on cigarette packets, should be printed on cassette headphones and displayed at entrances to discotheques. Young people would then be aware of the risks. At the moment, it is argued, they are being used as unsuspecting guinea pigs, as commercial music operators see how far they can go before the law—or public revulsion—intervenes.

The many case histories of youthful lives spoilt in this way make a grim catalogue. A student nurse attended a disco in, paradoxically, her hospital, and has since had screaming and metallic banging inside her head. Several sixteen-year-olds have been allowed to sit their school exams wearing headphones and listening to soft music intended to distract them from tinnitus. One twenty-five-year-old has never been able to work because of his injury caused at the age of thirteen when he stood too close to a powerful microphone at a family disco party. These are just a few examples.

Education in recent decades has taken on a cautionary role for children. Teachers tell first-year infants that they must not cross the road without looking and older boys and girls are warned about the hazards of drugs, solvents or

# DISCO DANGER LEVEL
## when pop music can
## give life-long head noise

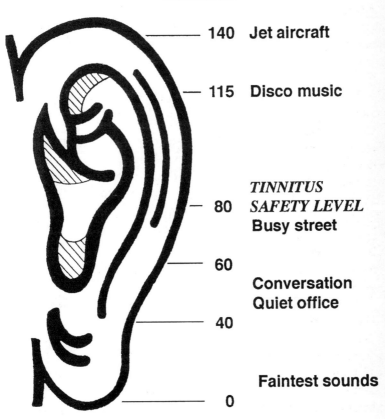

### Decibels

——— 140 **Jet aircraft**

— 115 **Disco music**

— 80 *TINNITUS SAFETY LEVEL* **Busy street**

——— 60 **Conversation Quiet office**

——— 40

**Faintest sounds**

——— 0

*Source:* **The British Tinnitus Association**

unprotected sex. Yet amid all this hardly a word is said about taking care of their precious sense of hearing—and the treasures of internal silence.

Without diminishing the value of other advice, it should be appreciated by parents and teachers that the statistical risk of getting tinnitus is greater than that for Aids, road deaths or unwanted pregnancies. While countless parents of stricken teenagers with permanent head noises regret that they did nothing to persuade their children to take care of their ears as well as the rest of their bodies, the voice of school-based authority remains silent. There is no formal provision for including tinnitus in classroom health education. Neither the Department of Education nor the local education authorities recognise the problem for the millions of young people for whom they have a responsibility. Such is the general indifference among teachers, that schools blithely organise end-of-term discos where the sounds, though not quite in the category of the club disco or rock concert, will edge into the real danger zone of 90-plus decibels and threaten health. In the absence of any official action by education leaders, some local tinnitus self-help groups have taken the initiative and supplied schools with teaching packs to explain what tinnitus is and how young people can to some extent protect themselves. One difficulty is convincing youngsters that tinnitus, so closely associated with deafness in some minds, is not confined to pensioners with hearing-aids.

While pop music boasts of creating aptly-named walls of sound, the safety warning is that it is dangerous to hit one's head against a wall, real or sonic.

As with many other medical conditions, both nurture and nature are said to be the cause of tinnitus. If toddlers can tell their parents about it, does the cause go back further to the process of birth or during the baby's time in the womb?

Many forms of deafness are known to be hereditary. As the onset of hearing loss and tinnitus can be experienced simultaneously at any age, can tinnitus be inherited? There are few statistics to support the belief that it can be. Moreover, as the scientific cause of head sounds itself remains seemingly light years from discovery, a convincing case cannot yet be made out that heredity has anything to do with it. It could be that a weakness in the intricate auditory system, which is considered less remarkable when it occurs in old age, is simply the premature fate of a child. The wide and still vague label of 'nature' can therefore be attached to infant cases, to await further explanation.

And does it start in the womb? For years people with good hearing and an even better memory have told how they can recall the steady sound-sensations of their own heart beats before birth. This cannot easily be dismissed as pure imagination, as a baby in the first minutes of life has a brain able to function on a basic level. It has been proved that babies are responsive to sounds before birth. Was it therefore vulnerable to loud noises which perhaps threatened its cosy safety and physically disturbed its hearing mechanisms, causing early tinnitus? If so, could, for instance, the raised voices of arguing parents, or a radio turned up too loudly, be blamed? As with so many areas of tinnitus study, there is no proof that this occurs, but the idea is attracting serious research in Belgium and France.

When a stricken child reaches school age the problems multiply. She has probably by then more or less adapted to the condition in her own way, maybe unaware that most people are without it. In the challenging environment of school she soon finds that she is different from her new friends. The psychological stress this can create, to say nothing of trying to hear what a teacher is saying while coping with her own sounds, call for expert handling in the form of child counselling. At the same time, teachers have to guard against slowness in learning caused by tinnitus being taken as a sign of lack of intelligence. The young sufferer faces a lifetime of handicap. She needs to have parents and teachers able to grasp, as well as any non-sufferers can, the unrelenting burden even the youngest may be called upon to bear.

# 2 Looking for Relief

Family doctors are known to display a brutal or casual streak when talking to a patient who has just experienced the start of tinnitus. 'Just learn to live with it.'—'Think about something pleasant.'—'Try to forget about it.' Millions of people who have gone to a surgery confidently expecting at least a prescription for relief, or reassurance that the noise will soon go away, have left devastated with the truth and shocked that a doctor with answers to in-growing toenails and headaches has nothing but the broadest type of advice. How can anyone forget such an intrusive complaint that is about as acceptable as a burglar in the living room? Especially if the intruder is screaming in the manner of tinnitus itself. Fear of the stranger, however, would greatly diminish if the surprised householder realised that he was harmless and had no intention of taking anything. And does a person with toothache continue to feel the pain when suddenly discovering his house is on fire?

If the mind can modify or dismiss the most acutely felt sensations of fear and pain, is it not fair to assume that tinnitus can be equally despatched from one's consciousness? I wish it could be, is the chorus answer of the tinnitus population.We think it can be, say a growing number of counsellors, therapists and researchers.

The pace towards this kind of treatment has been quickened by the experimental work and recent claims of one London researcher, Jonathan Hazell. His hopeful message, which has attracted attention throughout the world, is that sufferers can be trained to 'walk away' from and 'lose the perception' of tinnitus. The mixed reaction to this has ranged from sheer disbelief and disparagement to grateful endorsement.

Hazell, a fine surgeon with a role in both public and private medicine, understands the ear but also realises the limitations of the operating theatre. Indeed, the scalpel remains useless as a weapon against tinnitus, though many who suffer badly would willingly sacrifice their hearing if the noises could be taken away as well. Even if that were possible, total deafness would be an extremely high price to pay. Non-surgical methods must therefore offer the most hope, and the best of them, Hazell believes, lies in training people to use their own thoughts as a path to relief. His ground-breaking work is being conducted at a small research unit, which he heads, at the Middlesex Hospital in London, in conjunction with the nearby Royal Ear Hospital. 'We have come a long way and we are on the right track,' he told the startled but delighted tinnitus world in 1993.

In an article published in *Quiet*, the quarterly journal of the British Tinnitus Association, he explained:

Although the inner ear is often implicated in the generation of tinnitus, it is not with our ears that we hear sounds, but with the auditory subcortex situated near the surface of the brain's temporal lobe. Sounds take almost one third of a second to reach our subconsciousness after leaving the inner ear and during this time pass through a network of millions of nerve cells (neuronal networks), part of the most sophisticated computerised mechanism known to man! It is this system which allows us to extract tiny, but important, messages from the hurly-burly of everyday environmental sounds. It is this mechanism which allows a conductor of a symphony orchestra to tell which of the violinists is playing out of tune, while the tone-deaf young man sitting in the audience cannot tell whether he is listening to an orchestra or a brass band.

Hazell's team, which keeps in regular touch with an American neuroscientist engaged in parallel pioneering work in Maryland, has been finding out whether distressed patients might have had different 'listening training' to account for their problems. At the same time it has been necessary to look back into the evolutionary process of hearing and the functions of the brain and ear.

It is believed that as Man and his senses evolved, the need to identify threatening noises, such as those from predators, shaped the hearing process. Tiny signals picked up by the inner ear are selected by the neuronal networks in the brain, magnified and then perceived as loud noise. Early humans gradually learned to fear or hate such amplified sounds, in order to respond quickly to their threatening source. The stress of tinnitus triggers a similar mechanism. Hazell's team has therefore been trying, with some success, to find ways of retraining the thought processes of sufferers, changing common belief about the negative properties of tinnitus. It is already claimed that the treatment can remove the perception of tinnitus entirely for some, so that they no longer hear it.

Hazell further explained:

> The training programme also uses therapeutic wide-band noise (WBN) at a very low level . . . WBN seems to 'reset' the errant neuronal switches and permanently reduce tinnitus perception. We are also measuring the relationship between threatening beliefs about tinnitus and changes in tinnitus annoyance. Just as the conductor is trained to detect the sound of the errant violinist, we are retraining the neuronal networks so that they are no longer detecting the unwanted sound of the tinnitus signal coming from the ear.

Interest and hope among researchers and sufferers throughout the world will have also been raised by a part of Hazell's studies which looks beyond the ear and brain. It involves the efferent nervous system which controls many of our basic functions, from heart beat and breathing to muscle tension and adrenaline release. The efferent nerves controlling part of the ear could be an important element in the cause of tinnitus. By tracing activity in these nerves as patients undergo various kinds of therapy, it is hoped to discover which patients can benefit from a particular approach. And once doctors can control the efferent system selectively by means of drugs, they may be able to relieve tinnitus.

It is easy to imagine the problem as the ear itself containing the physical source of sounds. With the din sometimes resembling such tangible items as a whistle, drill or hammer, it is natural to believe that there is something equally touchable just inside the head giving rise to it all. Hazell warns: 'Unfortunately this gives a totally false picture of tinnitus from a scientific point of view. The reality is that tinnitus generators are very tiny and minute, barely measurable by our most sensitive laboratory techniques, even though tinnitus perception is very loud and distressing. The perception, however, is quite real, not in any way imagined, and will one day be measured.' The real power in the hearing mechanism comes from the central processing which is capable of amazing feats of signal detection and amplification. His concluding message when reporting on the work of his team was quite optimistic:

We are hopeful that one day we will be able to interfere with these brain mechanisms using drugs and even surgery, as well as do things to alter the generators. At the moment, the most effective approach is one which many people would label as 'psychological'. However, we believe that we have come a long way . . . We are not simply training people to tolerate their tinnitus, we are training the auditory pathways to change the pattern recognition involved in detecting tinnitus and to eliminate the perception of tinnitus. Although we do not achieve this with all our patients . . . the fact that it

is achieved at all means that we are on the right track.
For the first time we are able to say that a previously
well-established perception of continually annoying
and distressing tinnitus can be turned off.

Is psychological conditioning the best—maybe the only—
chance anyone has of finding a cure? Is being taught to reduce
the sounds to a minimum the only realistic hope to which
sufferers can cling? Critics of Hazell's findings say too much
is being read into results involving a small number of people.
Hopes could be cruelly raised on the basis of insufficient
evidence available. And is it feasible to construct a whole
new field of treatment on something which demands a highly
personalised contribution from the patient, namely the training of each unique mind and personality to achieve welcome
but subjective relief?
    There is certainly no shortage of volunteers keen to try
the retraining techniques, but no practicable arrangements
are possible for more than the tiniest fraction of them to join
the specialised course now running in London and a few
other clinics. For the foreseeable future, then, the treatment,
promising though it is, is a tantalising but unobtainable
prospect. Doubts, meanwhile, remain. For badly stressed
sufferers, their noises are just too loud and pervasive for
them to walk away from them. By and large they pin their
hopes on drugs or surgery, at some future date.

## SELF-HELP

'I've tried my GP, seen a specialist and even sampled some
of the alternative medicines. Now what shall I do?'
    That sums up the thoughts of many people when they
realise they have a permanent problem without solution.
The vast, collective wisdom of the world of medicine
cannot lead them to a quiet head. The chemist's shop, the
family doctor's surgery, the specialist's consulting-room,
the operating theatre, the hospital ward are all useless.

A Nobel Prize awaits some researcher, perhaps as yet unborn, who comes up with the answer—or one of many answers—to the question of how to cure tinnitus. But for the moment—or, more truthfully, for the indefinite future—the paramount question in the mind of the sufferer is: how can I lighten my burden by my own efforts?

Sooner or later, some sort of solution presents itself.

Nothing irritates more than a doctor's off-hand 'You'll just have to learn to live with it.' Such advice can sound facile, as if will-power is all that is needed to accommodate tinnitus and that perceived suffering is a sign of weakness and lack of personal grit. Yet it can be useful, if interpreted with a patient, open mind.

After all, not even the worst head noises make their presence felt every moment of the day. It may not be possible to banish them at will, but somehow they go into hiding for indeterminate periods of minutes or hours, when they are simply not heard consciously. No physical reason can be detected for these periods of transient relief. The sufferer is just happily but inexplicably unaware of his invisible companion. Is there an explanation? It is now apparent that the remission is due to the brain being so captivated by what the sufferer is doing that distraction and delight combine to put the tinnitus to flight—even if it is on a return ticket.

Direct advice on what to do to obtain such blessed distraction is as difficult and absurd as trying to tell anyone why they should prefer blue to yellow or a beech tree to an oak. It is no surprise to find, therefore, that anyone who can forget his tinnitus for a time has a near-bespoke recipe. What he recommends may not be unique, but it is probably different from the next person's ideas.

'I get great relief being out of doors,' said a middle-aged accountant who scarcely strayed away from his desk and his city flat before his noises started at the age of thirty-two. 'Now I sometimes think I would be better off living in a tree-house or the jungle. Being indoors magnifies the racket.'

He was voicing a common experience. In the largest of rooms, the four walls have the effect of a sound-box. Outside—whether in a quiet garden or a noisy street—the problem lessens. Many of the tinnitus population have discovered this.

One schoolteacher found both the class-room and the staff-room increased his tinnitus. The bliss of work out of doors beckoned, and he took a job labouring in the council's parks department, sometimes putting down the white lines on playing fields used by his former pupils. It was the best career move he was ever likely to make, for his health.

Conversion to the outdoor life does not always require such a drastic act, of course. It can entail spending more time in the garden, with often the bonus of a finer lawn and better-tended flower beds. Indeed, closer attention to plant life and the gardener's rejoicing in the intricacies and simplicities of all that a garden has to offer can provide a psychological antidote to the discordant horror going on inside the head, where nature seems to have lost her balance and decency.

Nature beyond horticulture has further curative or relieving properties. A high wind, for instance, can both drown tinnitus and give a caressing massage to the ears and head generally.

From waiting for the wind to whistle about your ears it is a small step to creating similar conditions—by moving quickly in the open air. The obvious ways to do this are by running, cycling or driving in an open-top vehicle. All these pursuits have been adopted with good effect by sufferers. A thirty-year-old man in Norfolk who never gave athletics a thought in school took up jogging and running in his late twenties and surprised himself by making rapid club-standard progress in a pastime he had approached purely as a relief from his sounds.

Running also brings generally improved health and a stronger physique, making a person somehow better equipped to deal with and minimise the feeling of ill health tinnitus brings for many. The same is true of cycling, which can make a person feel fitter as well as providing the undoubted therapy of having air rushing past the ears. Because of their greater speed, motorcycles are frequently favoured as a source of instant therapy. There are cases of people in their fifties climbing on to motorcycles for the first time in their lives, and revving away to find another weapon with which to fight their condition.

As taking to the road is just not feasible—either in running shoes or on a saddle—for much of the tinnitus population, it is fortunate that there are many other well-trodden paths to relief. They are almost as numerous as the people seeking them.

Tinnitus, with its capacity to flood the conscious mind, can sooner or later prompt the thought that the brain desperately needs other and new challenges.

It is a fair guess that many of the people who sign up for local adult education classes each autumn are, in part, really enrolling for tinnitus therapy. Painting, drawing, languages, keep-fit and other subjects certainly have their attractions. At their lowest level, they take people out of the house on regular evenings and away from the strains that tinnitus can create for all the family. More positively, they give a diverting outlet for minds bombarded day and night by unwelcome sounds.

It is even claimed by some sufferers that artistic expression, in writing, music or the visual arts, is the only adequate way of describing tinnitus to people without it. A drawing or painting of a tortured face silently pleading for quietness says more than the standard definitions found in medical dictionaries. A poem about what it feels like to lose silence for ever is more eloquent than what the average doctor can say about a tinnitus patient. The colours of an oil painting depicting inner torment can vividly represent the perpetual frustrations of the sufferer artist. If it deserves any gratitude at all, tinnitus can be thanked for stimulating a wealth of art which enables many people to find liberating relaxation in a world of inner sounds which sometimes seem capable of engulfing them.


## IN THE MIND

If being told 'to learn to live with it' by a doctor sounds less than helpful, an explanation that it is 'all in the mind' can be downright cruel. It is tantamount to telling a serious sufferer that the whole condition is imagined and can be defeated with will-power and determination.

The trouble springs from the age-old confusion of the words 'brain' and 'mind'. The brain is certainly involved in tinnitus and possibly is the source of it, as well as generating all thought and experience. It therefore shapes our mind. In tinnitus, therefore, the mind cannot be ignored when relief is sought. What annoys the sufferer is the slightest suggestion that the sounds can somehow be told to go away. Would that they could! Attitudes to one's own tinnitus are tremendously important, however, and can tip the balance between accepting head sounds and being defeated by them. The right frame of mind can reduce the perception of them.

The role of the psychologist is growing in importance and providing a lifeline to many who would otherwise have despaired. In some hospitals psychology plays a formal part in tinnitus treatment—either in a dedicated clinic or in an ENT department dealing mainly with deafness. It has much to do. Up to half of the patients can be expected to be distressed, variously irritable, depressed, angry, tense and anxious. These emotional problems have been quantified as the commonest effects of tinnitus, followed by difficulties in separating sounds (particularly voices) and insomnia. Interestingly, such effects can have an uneven pattern. A slightly anxious person, for instance, may be an insomniac, but someone with great anxiety may sleep deeply.

In spite of these facts, most of the tinnitus population manage to stop paying too much attention to the condition and it becomes less of a problem. This is called habituating to tinnitus. Research shows that habituation follows the same path as the process of getting used to anything potentially threatening or worrying, but in the case of tinnitus, progress can be slowed or halted if the sounds change, a person is very tense (sometimes due to other stresses) or emotional significance or meaning is attached to the tinnitus.

For psychological treatment to have any hope of success, relaxation has to be achieved; a truth discovered at home by sufferers, who universally find that tension and worry can worsen their noises, or how they perceive them. No less important, but rather more difficult, is changing their ideas on the very meaning of tinnitus. A good psychologist is well aware that tinnitus can create many differing beliefs and emotions, not always corresponding to the intensity of the noises. Often people believe from the start that it is a natural part of the ageing process and no strong emotions are aroused. Equally commonly, there is a collection of fears standing in the way of recovery. Beliefs leading to stress are catalogued under such headings as 'I must have a more serious illness', 'I cannot cope and will go mad', 'It isn't fair I have this', etc. The distress itself can distort a persons's belief about tinnitus and, in a vicious circle, perpetuate the distress.

Whether relaxation or cognitive therapy is used, success has been recorded. When patients are asked to describe the loudness of their tinnitus, they give roughly the same answers before and after the treatment. But they also say how they are less annoyed by it.

Do not be afraid or sceptical of psychological treatment any more than you would be of more tangible medicine following, say, an accident. If it is not offered, and you feel your state of mind could, as it were, do with a second opinion outside yourself, ask for it. Remember the skills of clinical psychologists can be applied to many conditions and distresses. They have encountered them many times in medical problems outside tinnitus, as well as in it. Your co-operation in this branch of healing could change your state of mind and show you that tinnitus is not half the monster it appears.

## IS IT WORSE THAN TOTAL DEAFNESS?

The whole subject of tinnitus, vast and extending into the outer reaches of human thought and back through history, is full of isolated and interlocking mysteries for the layman and scientist interested in it. What is the biggest conundrum, apart from questions of its future cure? Oddities and contradictions abound. Sufferers ask such things as 'Why do some people find the sound of a noisy party drowns it out, but it makes it worse for me?' Or 'How is it that a few drinks can partly blot out tinnitus in some people but one glass of red wine makes mine sound even more?' The contradictions are surely embedded in each person's unique nature and personality, both of which reflect their perception of tinnitus and their differing reactions to a common stimulus. It may not be a bad thing that tinnitus does not have fixed patterns in everyone. Without such uniformity, an individual can at least take some therapeutic interest in what is best for him, and take some comfort and hope from knowing to some extent what to do and not to do for his own special sounds. These personal contradictions, if indeed they deserve the name, can happily remain as mysteries on the unsolved list for as long as sufferers need to shape their habits and social activities in order to find a measure of peace.

Sufferers often ponder a common contradiction concerning deafness and tinnitus. Before very long after the inception of his sounds, the person experiencing tinnitus puzzles over the fact that someone with a lot of tinnitus can have very sharp hearing, but mild tinnitus can bring deafness.

A brief answer is that it is no more strange than the fact, which is accepted without question, that a severely deaf person does not necessarily have tinnitus. Surgeons and physicians point out that gradual ageing of or damage to the inner ear can cause hearing loss and noises at the same time but there is no scientific reason to expect the two things always to coincide. Moreover, slowly developing deafness is not always noticed until tinnitus starts, though the person swears they both started together. All of this is true but still does not provide us with the full explanation. Any extraneous noise can obliterate some sounds for anyone with good hearing. The brain learns—or is born with the ability—to separate sounds and hear, unimpaired, that which it needs to hear. But is there anyone who, say, listening to a string quartet would not be distracted or slightly 'deafened' by a baby suddenly screaming nearby? How, then, can serious tinnitus yell or drum away not nearby but right inside the head, and still not deafen? The most careful research to date in the brief two decades of scientific work on tinnitus still paints with too broad a brush to create an accurate picture of the brain/ear connection and its millions of components. The truth about deafness and tinnitus may one day be revealed in one swoop or painfully slowly, showing that the subjects have, after all, more distance between them than common ground. One can find dedicated researchers ready to embrace either view—or say it is too early to make an educated guess.

Sufferers and their families long to see tinnitus acknowledged in its own right, and universally seen as a serious problem pleading for undivided attention. Only then can there be adequate resources and dedication to tame and then destroy it. Thoughts on those lines remain somewhat wishful to date, but a start has been made in reaching the oft-stated goal. Meanwhile, deafness and tinnitus, even for those with head noises and no hearing loss, are bound to co-exist in the public's mind, as they do in researchers who believe that the conquering of deafness will also stop unwanted sounds. While they remain so closely linked, comparisons of the two conditions are inevitable. It is often asked which is the worse? To make any sense of the question, let alone answer it, one has to eliminate comparing an extremely bad example of one with a mild case of the other. Yet such an elimination is itself tricky, as there is no proper way of applying the same method of measurement to both. A technician can quickly plot the quantity and nature of someone's deafness in a test lasting a few minutes, while tinnitus remains resolutely subjective. The sufferer can equate given internal sounds to the frequency and volume of external sounds created for comparison, but his reaction to and tolerance of the tinnitus make up a crucial factor definable solely in terms, as yet objectively unexpressed, of his anguish or acceptance. Is there, then, any way to strike a comparison between the unpleasantness of totally deaf isolation and the ever-pervading presence of head sounds? The best way to find out, for the time being, is to listen to the spontaneous comments and anecdotal evidence of ordinary men and women through the years. What have they told their doctors, their friends and relatives? The most significant pointer may be the many times patients will ask if there is an ear operation to take away tinnitus, even if it meant losing their hearing totally. Such a question is naturally asked mostly by those with very bad tinnitus. The prospect of being rid of the sounds overcomes the thought of losing one's hearing. Their disappointment is great on being told that no such surgery is possible, and that operations on the ear can even worsen tinnitus. Equally significant in the quest for a true tinnitus/deafness comparison, there seem to be no instances of a deaf person wanting the reverse to happen. A totally deaf patient would never seriously ask for an operation to restore hearing if the inevitable price would be a mixture of loud permanent noises in the head. 'Cure my tinnitus and I'll willingly surrender my remaining hearing' is the cry from a large sample of the tinnitus population, of whom the worst sufferers have no difficulty in nominating deafness as the lesser affliction. Moreover, there simply does not seem to be a remotely acceptable way of measuring them alongside each other.

Broad public attitudes displayed by people with one or both of the conditions also throw up a chasm of perception between them. The hearing world would be surprised to learn of the strong advocacy of deaf culture among the deaf. Their loss of good, or any, hearing has led many to embrace their handicap not as something to be rejected as quickly as possible if cures are found but as a valued dimension in their whole lives. They speak of what they would miss if their hearing problem was solved. Among the perceived advantages is the loose network of deaf clubs, societies and contacts which have over the years enriched and sustained their lives. They value the comradeship and the social cohesion established among many deaf people and their helpers, including medical people and social workers. What, if anything, would be a suitable substitute if such unquantifiable bonuses were lost? And why should it be expected, they argue, that unalloyed joy would flood into their lives when good hearing would bring the noisy pollution of everyday life, with the high decibels of heavy traffic and perhaps noisy neighbours invading the enforced silence of deafness to which many have become accustomed? All this is not to say that deafness is not a horrible burden from which millions long to be relieved. The phrase 'deaf culture' is, none the less, increasingly on the lips of an articulate minority of deafened people who actually see at least some aspects of the deaf world which are positive, and certainly are not capable of being surrendered without very mixed feelings.

It is not easy to find people with deafness *and* tinnitus wishing to preserve the world as they experience it. The 'culture' of deafness does offer such people a safety net of local clubs and social contacts, in cases where they feel their afflictions would otherwise totally isolate them. Welfare for deaf people in an organised form stretches back well into the nineteenth century and provides understanding and support, even a purpose in life. But take away the handicap and its palliatives would soon become redundant, seems to be the general opinion of dual deaf-tinnitus sufferers. Some of them share the view of many disability groups that it is better not to hope and wait for a cure but to accept the reality and seek the best possible life within the unavoidable constraints. But attaching the word 'culture', even in its correct meaning, will never sanctify an essential unpleasantness or raise it to a way of life to be defended against what science and human progress may have in store. Still less likely is the prospect of much advocacy of 'tinnitus culture' on its own. The affliction does draw people together, among those who wish to meet socially on a regular club basis. The contacts and friendships thus gained in tinnitus groups are highly valued in their own right. People of all ages find the mutual support can give them the will to carry on with their lives and bear their tinnitus with hope and fortitude. It is good that such groups thus diminish the threatening potential of tinnitus, but they would require an attitudinal quantum leap to emulate some deaf people and talk about, with affection, their 'tinnitus culture'. This, then, is another way of showing that deafness and tinnitus, though often shared, are worlds apart. Its very rejection of 'culture' perhaps serves to indicate that tinnitus brings a suffering worse than that which total silence can bestow.

## FAMILY SUPPORT

'It was only when tinnitus started to creep into our everyday living that life went from bad to worse. It became the monster in our house.' Without knowing it, a Cheshire woman spoke for millions of people across the world when she described tinnitus in a family. Parents, spouses, siblings initially fail to grasp the seriousness of it all when they are told about it. The chances are that they have never heard of the condition or, having heard a few transient buzzings of their own, think it will go away. When the stress and torment become apparent, they feel mystified by the invisible intruder and then frustrated by their helplessness and inability to lessen the burden. Though no one can experience or share another's tinnitus, its ghastliness can easily spread. The whole family can be affected vicariously.

The woman's dilemma was deeply personal, but typical in its relentless intensity. 'My husband has had tinnitus for fourteen years along with hearing loss of approximately thirty decibels. When it first entered our lives it was mainly the deafness that caused the problem, with the children having to repeat things all the time and the volume of the television having to be turned up too loud for us', she said. 'I don't think that I really appreciated the effect it had on my husband. His noises were overwhelming some days and it was all he could do just to get up in the morning. He tried everything on the market to make his life more tolerable. It began to be a search for the miracle cure. By now all the children had left home and so I was the only one left to be the "sounding board". Some days the only relief my husband could get was to take a sleeping pill and go to bed. I have known him to sleep for over forty-eight hours. Me? I just have to sit and wait for him to return to the land of normality and be there for him with whatever I can say or do.

'Our social life is non-existent because of his tinnitus and deafness. We both like concerts but cannot go because they are too loud. Motor-racing is out. We both love going on holiday but the flying makes his ears so painful and the noises so bad that it just isn't practicable. Our grandchildren have to be careful not to shout, and certain DIY jobs are out because the noise level is too great. Research must be of paramount importance and the only way we will get enough is for us all to make as much "noise" about tinnitus as possible.'

In the wealth of good advice thrown up by the professionals and amateurs in the burgeoning world of self-help, there has not been much of practical value for the family. Relatives are expected to adapt to the situation and muddle through the domestic minefields of depression, anxiety and insomnia of the sufferer close to them. Human resilience, in all its

marvellous forms, however, is sometimes no match for the
mounting and endless misery. Advice from a person outside
the family can easily earn the response 'It is more easily said
than done.' In any case, how can there be general rules for
stressed families, no two of whom are alike or face exactly
the same situations, apart from a common irritant?

Eileen Hewitson, who helps to run the large Birmingham
and District Tinnitus Group and understands both the importance and practice of relaxation, has constructed a down-to-
earth programme already benefiting some of her members
and their families. She has told them: 'It is not easy being an
onlooker. It is sometimes very hard for non-sufferers to
understand what is going on. If you feel frustrated by your
inability to help, just put a little distance between yourself
and the sufferer for the time being. Try not to show your
frustrations to the one you are trying to help, as this could
make him feel guilty about spoiling your enjoyment. Try to
keep a sense of humour. Try to laugh with, not at, the
sufferer. Laughter is a great healer.' She lists the following
ten suggestions:

1   Try to be supportive and don't expect progress to be
    rapid. Learning to cope does take time. Remind the
    sufferer of this.
2   Try not to reproach the sufferer for spoiling your life.
    This can create extra anxiety.
3   Discuss your feelings about the problem. Talk posi-
    tively, trying to find ways to resolve your differences.
4   Try not to allow your own life to become seriously
    disrupted. It's one thing to miss a night out in the pub,
    it's another to stop seeing family and friends because
    the sufferer finds it difficult. This may cause you to
    become resentful of the sufferer and this resentment
    could become a problem in itself.
5   Sufferers need reassurance that they are still loved. This
    is very important because it is easy to lose confidence. A
    squeeze of the hand or a little hug can work wonders.

6 Try to give praise when the sufferer makes progress. Don't criticise lack of progress—sufferers know themselves when they are not coping very well.

7 Try not to make the sufferer feel an outsider. Keep inviting friends and family round and going out, even if it's been difficult before. This will remind the sufferer what to aim for.

8 Try to encourage new pursuits, hobbies and interests, especially if old ones are no longer so enjoyable.

9 Notice when the sufferer seems better, more his or her old self, and see if there is a pattern. Is the tinnitus less of a problem after exercise, after watching a comedy programme, a film, a nature programme, after a period of relaxation, a day out, listening to music, etc?

10 Self-help groups exist to support you as well, so attend meetings, read newsletters. Find someone you can talk to about your side of the problem. A trouble shared is a trouble halved.

It is difficult to describe tinnitus to someone else, and this problem has been recognised by the Nottingham Tinnitus Clinic. In their written advice to new patients, they tell non-sufferers:

> One way to get some idea of what your relative or friend is suffering is to tune a radio off-station until a constant whining sound can be heard. Then ask the person with tinnitus to adjust the volume control so that the whine has the same loudness as his tinnitus. Then leave the radio on beside you all evening, especially when you want to relax or go to sleep or are reading the paper.
>
> What should you do about it? The tinnitus patient's main need is for better understanding of the problem by family and friends, especially on those occasions when the tinnitus makes them get tense, irritable or depressed. The patient in turn must do everything he

can not to let the tinnitus make him a permanent invalid or misery, and not to take advantage of the family's sympathy.

Deafness is a common companion of tinnitus, and friends and relatives can help by understanding what it is like. The Nottingham Clinic advises:

Try putting on the television during a talk programme such as the news, and then turn the volume down so that it is difficult to hear. Then put on a radio, selecting a music programme and adjusting it to a level that is almost as loud as the sound from the television. Try listening to that. The difficulty you experience may be very similar to what your relative or friend experiences most of the time: the voice is not quite loud enough and it is difficult to distinguish each word clearly.

The person with both tinnitus and deafness (even fairly slight) can be immeasurably helped in his battle to cope if other people:

1   Speak slowly and clearly, without shouting.
2   Avoid long or awkward sentences.
3   Face the hearing-impaired person, in good light.
4   Keep their temper.
5   Do not decline to repeat something, by saying it was not important.
6   Speak one at a time.
7   Do not talk against a background of music or other broadcast sounds.

The value of lip-reading should not be forgotten. It is not widely appreciated that everyone 'reads' other people's lips, to some extent. Try closing your eyes when the newsreader is looking straight at the camera during a TV news broadcast and you will find it more difficult to hear what is being said. The tinnitus-deaf person will thank you if you:

1 Make sure your face can be seen properly in good light, avoiding standing with a bright light behind you.
2 Get the attention of the lip-reader before speaking.
3 Speak a little more slowly than usual, but do not exaggerate your lip movements, as this can be seen as a visual distortion.
4 Speak simply.

# 3   Mechanical Aids

The expanding use of gadgetry in the home has brought with it a bonus for anyone with tinnitus. The inventors and designers can be said to have succeeded in making unwanted noises less of a bother, where the medics have hitherto failed. It is true that many excellent and fairly inexpensive products are marketed with deaf people in mind, but they can be of real benefit to tinnitus sufferers with no hearing loss.

## GADGETS FOR THE HOME

In the controlled conditions of an audiology department a person with tinnitus may be found to have no deafness but in the conditions of everyday living, the distracting power of ceaseless internal noise can cause many of the disadvantages known to the deaf person, such as not hearing a door-bell or not being able to hear a television programme or radio properly. Almost without exception, devices made for the deaf are therefore of value to tinnitus people—more so, of course, if they are also deaf.

One portable door signal can provide chimes and flashing lights anywhere in the house or garden up to 50 metres from the front door and the system can incorporate up to four bell pushes to cover other doors. It is suitable for tinnitus sufferers who add to their anxiety by worrying that they will miss callers to the home. A TV or radio volume can be turned up without annoying anyone else in the room by using a personal infra-red system. A transmitter picks up the

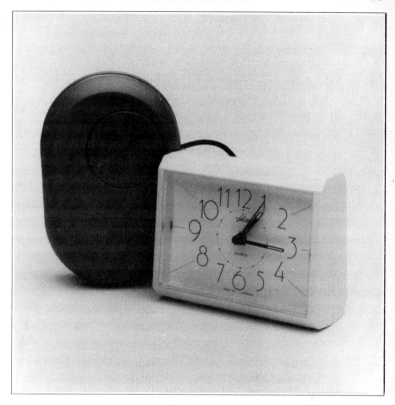

*Incoming telephone calls are signalled by this flashing light plugged into the phone and mains socket. It is bright enough to be seen in daylight, and is a help for deaf-tinnitus sufferers who find it difficult to hear even an amplified ringing signal.*

voices or music from the set and sends them via an invisible beam to a small receiver, from which it is possible to pick up the transmission with earphones or a hearing-aid. Another system uses hidden cables to form a domestic loop system, similar to those used in public halls and theatres. The deaf or tinnitus-distracted person listens to the broadcast by switching the hearing-aid to its 'T' position, and can control volume and tone, enjoying an intimate reception of the sound. No one else need hear the radio or TV, but can do so.

Tinnitus can be especially troublesome when a telephone is being used, somehow mingling with and distorting the speech of the incoming call. A portable amplifier can be fitted on to most phone receivers, with the option of producing a loop signal for use with a hearing-aid, if worn. Calls which may not be heard ringing are less likely to be missed when a small flashing device to indicate an in-coming call is used. Anyone unable to hear an alarm-clock can buy one with a pillow vibrator connected. Another alarm-clock on

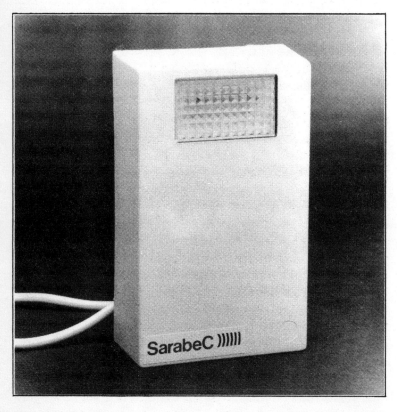

*If tinnitus and deafness cause you to miss the sound of an alarm clock, this powerful pillow vibrator can make wake you up on time. An audible signal is also produced.*

the market causes a reading-lamp to flash at a pre-set time.

Insomnia brought about by tinnitus can be defeated, strangely enough, with the help of extra sounds. A device is placed under the pillow and brings soothing tones to the person trying to sleep. The sound lasts for an hour before the volume gradually fades and switches itself off. Another more sophisticated device for sleep inducement involves a small ear-worn instrument picking up sounds from an induction pad under the pillow. The pad is linked to a radio, CD player or tape-cassette player, giving the tinnitus sufferer the choice of music or a tinnitus-masking tape made for the purpose. No one else can hear the sounds. Long before such devices were manufactured, the use of radio as a means of blocking out some of the tinnitus for sleepless people was widely recognised. People would—and some still do—go to bed with their ears connected to a portable radio or simply listening to the radio or TV, without earphones, turning off the set when they woke in the morning. Some recommend the method as a way of giving the subconscious mind something to listen to through the night instead of picking up the tinnitus and perhaps interrupting sleep by doing so.

Listening to recorded broadcast music or speech can call for added concentration if it is competing with constant sounds in the head. It can be made easier by wearing good quality headphones which totally cover the ears and preferably have separate volume controls on each side. By also adjusting the tone and treble/bass controls on the radio, TV (when the set permits) or stereo equipment, it is possible to produce varied signals to match the tinnitus or hearing loss in each ear. The headphones can also be used with the smaller kinds of internal hearing-aids, which themselves can incorporate adjustable tone and volume.

Less easily understood is an instrument which, when held near the ear, can be made to produce electromagnetic waves to relieve the tinnitus. Originally designed to treat muscular pain, it has since impressed some audiologists in a trial conducted in Liverpool. A few patients reported total remission and others said their sounds had lessened but others found no relief. If the harmless waves are partly beating tinnitus it is not known exactly how they are doing so. The total failure for many sufferers is thought to show that the gadget is effective only in respect of tinnitus springing from certain causes, but as the causes of tinnitus are still only a matter of speculation and cannot be categorised, the random success of the device, marketed as Therapak, is not a strong enough reason to dismiss it. Electromagnetism is a powerful force with a wide range of uses. One could well be the genuine defeat of some tinnitus.

The greater use of captioning has meant that millions of viewers with hearing problems can fully enjoy videoed programmes. For the captions to be read in the home a small adaptor can be purchased and plugged into the TV set. The combination of sounds in the head and even slight deafness can wreck normal TV watching, most of the speech being quite unintelligible. Thanks to the initiative of the National Captioning Institute, thousands of videos have been captioned and are among those available for purchase or hire in high streets.

Tinnitus can make visits to places of public entertainment less attractive, but the steady spread of technology means life at home can be made more tolerable.

## HEARING-AIDS

Along with artificial additions to the heart, keyhole surgery and laser treatment, the hearing-aid today represents a marvel of science and technology. The ear-trumpet of other centuries and the body-worn, cumbersome equipment provided in the early days of the National Health Service are now curious items in medical museums. The technology of miniaturised engineering has come to the rescue of millions of deaf people, enabling them to make the most of any hearing they still have.

Tinnitus, so close to, yet profoundly different from,

deafness in many ways, has become something of an accidental beneficiary of the dramatic improvements made in the design and manufacture of aids in recent decades. A person with tinnitus and quite a lot of hearing loss can benefit from wearing something that can amplify speech and other sounds to enable him to hear better. He can also have a sound-generating masker incorporated in the aid to blot out or distract attention from the tinnitus sounds. Fortunately the aid can additionally be of help to anyone with tinnitus but without deafness.

To understand how anyone with good hearing can find any use in having an aid in one or each ear it is necessary to know how countless sufferers manage to go through life putting up with the racket in their heads. Although most find they wish to avoid noisy places, total silence can increase the tinnitus. Various levels of sound between these two extremes can bring relief. Depending on the personality, the degree of tinnitus and perhaps other medical conditions, acceptable volume and type of sound can reduce the personal perception of internal noise. Music and speech thus become so important; a sufferer will often say, for instance, that buying enough radios to have one in every room in the house can be the best of all investments.

Except for those people with hypersensitive hearing, most uninvited sounds throughout the day are acceptable. The neighbour's lawn-mower, the passing bus, the bark of a dog are, in moderation, only indications of the world around us in which most people are content to play a role. The tinnitus sufferer, with his sounds intricately bound up as much with the brain as with the ears, seems subconsciously to find consolation in the sound of the world beyond his personal affliction. He is silently rejoicing that sound, so unwelcome when uninvitedly squatting in his head, still takes many benign forms in the world. With or without such philosophy, ambient sounds certainly have the power to make the tinnitus recede and lose its potency. And this is where a hearing-aid helps.

The NHS does not openly dispense hearing-aids solely to help tinnitus when a patient has no hearing loss. Where the deafness is quite slight a person can, however, find himself wearing an aid almost wholly to the advantage of his tinnitus and scarcely, if at all, to correct the deafness of which he may not even be aware. The aid slightly exaggerates the everyday sounds around him and thereby cuts back the conscious awareness of the tinnitus.

It is a matter of personal adaptation and trial and error to discover at what volume setting to use the aid in order to block the tinnitus. In a busy, noisy street the sound of traffic and pedestrians can actually assist and the lowest setting can often be chosen. In a quieter place like a park, a higher setting enhances the natural aural ambience, so checking the ill-effects.

Another category of sufferers—those with some deafness but not willing to admit it, saying that it is simply tinnitus blocking out clear conversation—can be agreeably surprised at what an aid can do for them. They may still maintain, quite inaccurately, that the improved hearing is because the aid is reducing the tinnitus. There is probably no harm in their misconception. There is undoubted benefit to be enjoyed in their better hearing and the anti-tinnitus effect of wearing an aid.

Where there is more deafness in one ear than the other (with or without tinnitus) the conventional and proven wisdom is to wear the aid in the better ear, contrary to what a newly deafened person may think. When the aid is primarily used as an anti-tinnitus device, as described above, the choice is not so straightforward. Head sounds can be experienced as if they are in one or both ears, or in neither and in the head generally. Unlike choosing the better ear in the case of deafness, it can be best to opt for the ear with the worse (or sole) sensation of tinnitus. If that one happens to be the deafer also, the use of two aids suggests itself, with different volume settings in each. If there is no noticeable deafness, but the tinnitus is somewhere in the middle of the head, it can be a matter of trying the aids separately in each ear and in both. For some there is a simple test of the anti-tinnitus properties of aids essentially made to help the deaf. The wearer should spend a little time in a busy street with the volume adjusted fairly low. Still close to the traffic, she should then quickly switch off the aid without first reducing the volume. The immediate result is not just reduced traffic noise but a brief but distinct increase in the tinnitus, as if it were keen to reassert its dominance once the enhancement of ambient sounds had ceased. After a second or two the tinnitus falls to its usual volume, but the person is left with proof that a hearing-aid can be a boon.

Assisting a partly-deaf person to hear is never just a case of speaking more loudly, though that helps. Good hearing involves the constant recognition, separation and perception of sounds of varying pitch, frequency and timbre, at great speed and largely without the conscious knowledge of the hearer. A piece of equipment that essentially amplifies sound is therefore of limited potential to either the deaf or the tinnitus-stricken, though better than nothing. The earlier aids and many in current use crudely act as amplifiers, and have not always matched up to the seemingly basic yet complex task of achieving a degree of aural normality. But the future is becoming brighter. It is misleading to talk of artificial ears; were they ever to be in reach, the brain could not be relied on to relinquish its mysterious part in the creation of tinnitus. Yet in the not-too-distant future hearing-aids could be as refined and sophisticated as any spare parts now being implanted routinely to compensate for malfunctioning organs in the body. They could be made by bespoke engineering tailored to an individual rather than the current off-the-peg equipment which still constitutes most of what is on offer. This will add to the masking qualities of aids and, for dual tinnitus-deafness sufferers, lighten the burden of deafness and enable them to fight their tinnitus more confidently.

The real hope of better things to come lies largely in highly specialised research being undertaken at Cambridge

University. A research team there is analysing the commonest causes of deafness and is already reporting with some confidence how distorted and diminished sounds reaching the ear can be corrected.

Most people's hearing loss is caused by damage to the sensory cells in the inner ear, which process incoming sounds of all sorts from a whisper to a clap of thunder. Their great virtue is having a mechanism referred to as automatic gain control (AGC) or compression which boosts weak sounds. This is lost in a deaf person. The threshold for detecting sounds is higher but the level at which sounds are uncomfortable stays the same. In these circumstances a conventional hearing-aid amplifies sounds equally so that when weak sounds are audible the louder sounds are uncomfortable. There is also a mechanism in normal ears which refines the selection of frequencies in complex sounds and enables speech to be understood, even when there is background noise. Hearing-aids are badly needed to incorporate signal processing and to compensate for any loss of the natural mechanism.

The Cambridge research team, which specialises in hearing-aids, has made possible the development of a prototype aid with three separate types of AGC, all of which is of real relevance to people whose tinnitus interferes with their hearing:

1 The first type adjusts the volume sensitively, so that the wearer can move from a quiet environment to a noisy one, without experiencing discomfort. The wearer does not have to adjust the controls.
2 The second control acts very quickly to protect a person from sudden loud sounds like china breaking or a door being slammed. The intervention is brief enough to deal with the sudden noise but without changing the sounds—perhaps voices—that follow.
3 The third, and most rapid, form of control is to enable a person to hear weaker speech sounds such as 'p' or 'k'.

It increases weak high frequency sounds, making speech more intelligible, especially in noisy situations.

Laboratory work is also proceeding to improve the degree to which amplification is matched to an individual's general needs at different frequencies. People who become deaf through age or loud noise have greater hearing loss at the high frequencies. It will be a great step forward when a standard hearing-aid reflects these different needs. New digital processing techniques will also one day make poss- ible greater hearing clarity and isolation of a single voice in a crowded room. Some of the more expensive hearing-aids sold privately already have some AGC and some pro- grammable aids have settings which adapt to different situations throughout the day. Advice on choosing an aid can be obtained from the London-based Hearing Research Trust (see address at end of book).

## MASKERS

Putting more sound into the head to reduce what is already there is, superficially, as crazy as trying to put out a fire with petrol. It is, however, the best means of relief for a minority of sufferers. The everyday sound of traffic, radios and the like all partly drown tinnitus or distract attention from it, so why not take suitable anti-tinnitus sounds right into the ears? The idea caught on in the 1970s, when the first ear-worn maskers were manufactured.

A masker is quite a small device with some big benefits. It can be either accommodated independently in the ear or as part of a hearing-aid. It simply makes a fairly neutral *sshhh* sound. The volume is controllable by the wearer but it does not change in pitch. For the luckiest it totally obliterates the tinnitus, although the masker's sound is still heard. It is comforting to know that this pleasanter experience is also generated mechanically from outside the head and can be controlled; it somehow creates a better environment and the

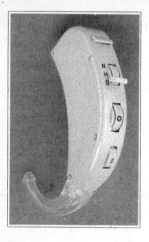

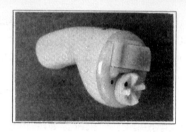

*A micro masker-only worn wholly inside the ear. From AudiMed of Beckenham, Kent.*

*A powerful behind-the-ear instrument combining a hearing-aid and tinnitus masker. From AudiMed of Beckenham, Kent.*

tinnitus seems less intrusive and troublesome.

For many people, maskers can be disappointing. They do nothing to reduce the loudness of tinnitus, and if a person is greatly troubled, the introduction of a soothing distraction often makes no difference. But the success stories include amazing claims of recovery. A masker rarely brings instant relief. Rather, the wearer must be prepared to persevere with it, in the nature of a protracted experiment, throughout the day for many months. Those who abandon it with impatience after a short while could be their own worst enemies. The extra sound, say some researchers, actually defeats or weakens tinnitus by a complicated route. Because of a malfunction of the auditory process, the brain exaggerates some otherwise slight sounds, including tinnitus, but is partly and safely desensitised by the continuous masking sounds, and therefore no longer amplifies the tinnitus signals.

Provision of free maskers under the NHS is patchy. In some ENT departments of hospitals there is not enough money to supply them to patients. In others there is little interest shown in them among medical staff, and it is quite common for them not to be mentioned to patients who could probably benefit from them. Outside the NHS, maskers are not very expensive to buy—nearer £50 than £100—and only a fraction of the price of a hearing-aid. They are obtainable from retail outlets normally selling hearing-aids or direct from a growing number of manufacturers, who will return most of the charge if the masker wearer is not satisfied with it after a few weeks.

A form of masking can be obtained without any special device. An FM radio tuned between stations can give the right *sshhh* sound to counter tinnitus. There are also small table-top devices giving a masking sound and some can be plugged into a pillow speaker to help a sufferer to sleep.

# 4   Professional Help

Everyone has experience, sooner or later, of being sent to see a specialist by their GP. This invariably means, in the NHS, an appointment with the medical or surgical head of a local hospital department, with subsequent treatment as an out-patient or admission for surgery. The consultant involved is, to the layman, the specialist, who is expected to dispense a cure or improvement in health. The picture for a tinnitus patient being referred to a 'specialist' is, alas, less clear.

For most of the population, the appointment is at an ENT (ear, nose and throat) department, in the absence of a tinnitus clinic. The man or woman in charge is, of course, an ear specialist with years of experience, but is he or she more or less equally qualified to deal with tinnitus? The ENT consultant will have been trained and specialised as a surgeon or a physician—a vital distinction for anyone innocently thinking that ENT departments everywhere are more or less equally geared up to treat them. A surgeon, marvellously skilled as he may be with the scalpel, is likely to have a lingering frustration when it comes to tinnitus. In only a very tiny number of cases can an operation help. He will also know, moreover, that occasionally an operation on an ear for any other purpose can actually cause or worsen tinnitus.

What chance does tinnitus have of receiving a fair hearing, so to speak, from a surgeon who can call upon the wonders of technology in the operating theatre to help him achieve astounding feats but who has to stand defeated when dealing with head noises? Being able to operate on the ear successfully counts for nothing. It is the surgeon ENT consultant, then, who is likely to say 'learn to live with it, there is nothing to be done', leaving the patient to face a comfortless future.

If the ENT head is a physician, on the other hand, a more helpful approach can be expected. He has probably built up a clinic with the wider range of skills needed to deal with the many side effects and consequences of tinnitus. The resulting sympathetic environment can do the patient an immeasurable amount of good.

It is largely pot luck whether your local specialist is a surgeon or a physician. Indeed you are unlikely to give the matter a thought while waiting for an appointment. Should you wish to, it is easy to consult the hospital's list of consultants, and see if the ENT person has the letters MRCP, FRCP or FRCS after his name (P is for Physicians, S for Surgeons). This is a rough and ready guide, as some surgeons are excellent when dealing with tinnitus and do not regard it as an annoying insoluble problem tacked on to the serious work of ear and deafness treatment. It could be the first step, though, if you wish to shop around and ask your GP to send you to a hospital where the specialist is likely to be tinnitus-friendly. In time the tinnitus-treatment distinction between the two categories of specialism will be eroded, to everyone's benefit. The first step will involve giving all medical students a greater knowledge of tinnitus during their general training, long before those who wish to specialise do so. Another change will be the gradual loss of autonomy for ENT heads, with policy-makers in hospitals and wider hospital authorities influencing the allocation of resources to tinnitus treatment.

## COUNSELLING

Advice to most patients consists of a few words in a busy GP's surgery or yet more hectic out-patients department of a hospital. It will probably involve drugs being prescribed or a proposed course of treatment and preventive strategies to avoid deterioration of a condition. With tinnitus, so hard to explain, let alone physically treat, is such advice enough? For anyone struggling to cope, especially soon after the onset of the noises, it is not. A relaxed, face-to-face dialogue is required and can best be provided by a trained counsellor.

Counselling is a developing profession rapidly winning its spurs. Qualified practitioners have undergone two years of training before becoming registered members of either the British Association for Counselling or the counselling section of the British Psychological Association. Tinnitus sufferers offered this help should remember that the present law allows anyone to call themselves a counsellor and sell their services. The amateurs are not necessarily to be avoided, but their professional counterparts think they should be known as lay-counsellors or helpers.

Do seriously consider any offer of counselling made to you. It may be suggested by a hospital specialist or a self-help tinnitus group in your town, but the intentions will be the same: to enable you to master your sounds. Unfortunately it is common for people to be too proud to admit that someone else can help them in this way. Sufferers from tinnitus often feel that they alone can manage, and their inner feelings are no one else's proper concern. If time is wasted because of this, negative attitudes towards the condition can become deeply embedded in the sufferer. Later, if counselling is accepted as a good idea, relief can be proportionately harder to find.

Resistance to accepting the advisory skills of others can best be conquered by knowing something of the qualities regarded as essential in a counsellor and how they can be used to the best advantage. (Indeed, a person with tinnitus most willing to receive counselling can also expect to get more from it by understanding the strengths of counsellors and how they hope to assist.) Helping a person by listening and talking is a nebulous skill but based on three

qualities: empathy, warmth and genuineness. A good counsellor should possess all three of them.

Empathy is seen as the ability to experience another person's world as if it were one's own without ever losing the 'as
if' quality. It is distinct from sympathy. It is 'about understanding another person's world irrespective of whether or
not emotional comfort is offered' according to Laurence
McKenna, a London psychologist with a special interest in
tinnitus. 'It does not involve judgement of the client. It is
about understanding what it is like to be the person in need of
help. A failure to communicate empathy may lead the client to
think that the counsellor does not understand or recognise
what he is going through, or does not care.'

The second quality to be noted in a good counsellor,
warmth, is respecting you for what you are, your individ-
uality and uniqueness in the human race. A climate must be
created in which anyone receiving help feels essentially
safe. To achieve this, the counsellor must fully accept you,
whatever your background or personality. You will soon feel
any warmth through the counsellor's active listening, sharing insights and valuing your opinions and feelings.

The final ingredient, genuineness, will certainly be absent
if the counsellor pretends to fill the role of a super-helper on
a plain above you. For it to work best she will try to
establish a relationship as with a working colleague on a
joint project or with a member of her family tackling an
issue of mutual concern. Don't be surprised if the counsellor
does not hide her own thoughts and feelings. This is seen as
beneficial, as long as the aim is to understand your inner
world and how tinnitus is colouring it.

Even the best planned and conducted course of interviews
will have its failures. If every other type of treatment has
been unsuccessful, it would be expecting too much to expect
counselling to bear fruit for everyone. On the credit side,
there are countless cases of people of all ages learning to
live with tinnitus in a manner they could not contemplate
before counselling. Undoubtedly some owe their lives to it.

## QUESTIONS AND ANSWERS

Often bewildered and frightened, or just irritated by their sounds, patients have plenty of questions for their GPs or hospital specialists.

Here are some of them and the answers they get:

### Migraine to Blame?

*I have had migraine for nearly twenty years and my tinnitus, which started fairly recently, always seems worse when I have a migraine attack. Should I blame the migraine, or the drug I take to relieve it, for the tinnitus?*

You are probably right to link your migraine with the tinnitus. There is a strong connection between the two. It is common for migraine sufferers to develop tinnitus later. If it is continuous tinnitus it can worsen during migraine. It has been found that the migraine drugs can reduce tinnitus in the same patient. This can happen where the tinnitus seems to replace migraine or gets worse during it.

### A Possible Trigger

*I developed glaucoma and tinnitus almost at the same time. The latter seemed to start when I used eye-drops for the former. Could it be just a coincidence? I also wonder whether my rheumatism has caused tinnitus. I am seventy-eight.*

The cause of tinnitus can only sometimes be identified. You mention three of the afflictions age can bring. Frequently two things can start together, or one starts as treatment is changed for the other. It is natural to wonder if they are linked. Head sounds starting in the elderly can very often be traced to the loss of sensitivity of the hearing system, which can be measured in a hearing test. A person does not always notice this as a deafness problem but it can certainly bring on tinnitus. Your tinnitus would have probably started anyway, but it is just possible that the glaucoma or migraine may have triggered the noises.

## Troubled Teenager

*My son is sixteen and about to sit his school exams. He is worried about coping with his tinnitus in the exam conditions as he notices it more in complete silence.*

The condition is rare among teenagers, but not unknown. People of all ages find it more troublesome in quiet surroundings. Your son should try wearing a sound masker in the ear to create a low level of background noise for himself. There is a danger that if he turns up the sound—which no one else will hear—to drown the tinnitus completely, the masking sound will annoy him just as much. He should try just taking the edge off his tinnitus. In rare cases students have been allowed to listen to music as a soothing diversion on their personal earphone stereos during examinations. Away from the examinations, many young sufferers find they can study best if they listen to soft music from a radio or cassette. It can partly submerge the tinnitus, and after a while they pay no attention to it or the music. The 'shsh' noise of a radio tuned off-station can also help in the same way.

## Treatment Danger

*Could an osteopath help me?*

If a neck disorder does not cause particular tinnitus, it can certainly make it worse. Both conditions can cause tension, which creates aches in the head or neck. So treatment of the neck has been known to help tinnitus, and osteopathy is one such treatment. In cases of continuous or recurring neck trouble it is worth thinking about osteopathy, but first consult your GP. It could just be harmful in certain fairly rare kinds of neck disorder.

## Are These Drugs Safe?

*I have heard that tinnitus can be started or worsened by diazepam (Valium) or any of the benzodiazepine drugs.*

No, it cannot. On the contrary, these drugs can be quite a help in managing tinnitus, producing a reduction in tension. If the tension has caused an increase in the noises, any reduction will also bring the tinnitus down. But there is always the problem of dependency, with patients finding it hard to stop taking these drugs after a time. When someone withdraws from them, especially if it is done rapidly, they can become anxious and tinnitus can result. Generally such tinnitus does disappear when the process of drug withdrawal finishes.

## Dizzy and Unbalanced

*Tinnitus has been with me for a long time and recently I have felt dizzy and cannot always stand up straight. I also have arthritis in the neck. Is it all connected?*

The inner ears receive their blood supplies via arteries each side of the spinal column in the neck. Arthritis can partly obstruct these arteries and this results in a reduction of the blood supply to the inner ears, where the organs of both balance and hearing are housed. The tension in the neck caused by the arthritis makes the whole condition much worse. Physiotherapy can be useful, but any relief is generally temporary. There are drugs which can diminish giddiness as well as improving blood circulation. Low-energy treatment on particular trouble spots such as the neck is in its infancy, but could help, just as deep heat therapy sometimes does.

## My Foot Problem

*As I believe some anti-fungal drugs can cause tinnitus, what should I do about my athlete's foot?*

When anti-fungal ointment or powder is applied to the infected area there is no risk of causing or aggravating tinnitus. If such treatment fails, a drug can be taken by mouth, but there are no reports of side effects from this either. The only drug known to affect hearing (and possibly tinnitus) is one sometimes prescribed for fungal infections connected with the bowel.

## Danger in this Hospital Noise?

*I am due to have a magnetic resonance imaging at a hospital and I am told the machine is very noisy. It is necessary to lie in it for some twenty minutes while scanning takes place. Do you think this will make my tinnitus worse? It is however important that I have the scan.*

It would be most unfortunate if a hospital examination, of all things, increased or created tinnitus, but the amount of noise involved in this scanning is not great and does not last dangerously long. Sometimes, however, a short burst of noise at a fairly low volume can trigger tinnitus in an ear which already has some disorder in it, caused perhaps by ageing, of which the person is not aware. Where tinnitus is already present, the sound of a scanning machine could just make it worse temporarily. To reduce that slight risk, ear-plugs could be worn. These can be purchased or made at home from cotton wool moistened with Vaseline.

## An Eastern Remedy?

*I have heard there is a possible remedy called* Ginkgo biloba. *Is it worth trying?*

This is an extract from the leaf of the Japanese maiden-hair tree and claims are made on its behalf in many countries. It can be bought in tablet form in health shops and has been tried for tinnitus in the UK without success for most people. A handful of sufferers say they have obtained some relief from it. The drug is not available on the National Health Service. It can be safely tried, and does not cost a great deal, but be prepared to be disappointed and do not expect a miracle.

## Cholesterol

*Did the cholesterol tablets I take cause my noises?*

It is highly unlikely. Your tinnitus and high cholesterol in your blood may be indirectly linked, but reducing the latter will not diminish the former.

## Blood Pressure Treatment

*I have taken various tablets for high blood pressure over the years and have found that some of them increase tinnitus. Can this be a cause and effect?*

The inner ear is not affected by such drugs, so they cannot be blamed. A small percentage of people find their tinnitus does get louder over the years, but generally not by a big margin. You could just be in this small statistical group, and changing your blood pressure tablets was only a coincidence.

## Dental Fillings

*Should I avoid having my teeth filled with mercury amalgam? I am told it can give you tinnitus, or in my case make it worse.*

Although any danger from this widely used dental amalgam has not been proved, mercury is recognised as a dangerous substance in many circumstances and fears about its use in the mouth are understandable. Various parts of the body can be adversely affected by mercury, and the ear cannot be totally excluded as a vulnerable organ. Tell your dentist about your tinnitus and any fear you may have of this type of filling. A dental drill can aggravate tinnitus, incidentally, so you may wish to use ear-plugs while in the dentist's chair, although these will probably not totally exclude the sound.

## Dentistry to Blame?

*My tinnitus started after receiving dental treatment, when I was also given an antibiotic to combat any underlying infection. Could any of this have caused my noises?*

It is possible for tinnitus and deafness to follow within a few hours of a visit to a dentist, but as this is so rare the link cannot be proved with statistics. The most likely explanation of your sounds is that the stress, which surrounds dental treatment for many people, triggered the problem. It is believed that stress can cause sounds when the hearing system is already damaged, but this damage can be so slight a person is quite unaware of it. It is unlikely that the antibiotic did it.

## Noisy Work

*If a noisy environment can cause tinnitus, can one ear only be affected?*

Noise nearly always brings deafness to both ears fairly equally, but if tinnitus also starts it can be in one or both ears, or seemingly in the middle of the head. The state of the ears before the damaging exposure to the loud noise can be a factor. If a disorder of one ear already exists, the volume of sound into that ear may be at a reduced level, and the risk of tinnitus lessened. The source of industrial noise can be nearer to one ear than the other through most of the working day, of course, but as it is reflected off walls it is unlikely to pose a greater threat to one ear than the other.

## Neck and Jaw Trouble

*I have read that pain and stiffness in the neck and jaw can have something to do with sounds in the head. Would treatment for them reduce the tinnitus?*

The connection has been suspected for many years. Surveys have shown that people with sounds are more likely to have neck or jaw and bite disorders. As is often the case in studying possible causes of tinnitus, however, it is hard to see how jaw and neck disorders can be connected with the inner ear. It is not much more than a guess, but the pain involved could send signals through the nervous system to the brain and create the perception of tinnitus. If arthritis of the neck is causing the pain, blood supply to the inner ear could easily be affected. Also, trouble in the neck and jaw can create muscular tension in the head, which is capable of aggravating tinnitus. Physiotherapy or osteopathy can do much to relieve stiffness and pain in and around the neck, and there are many claims that this can reduce the tinnitus.

## Beethoven's Tinnitus

*I read that Beethoven had otosclerosis. Did it cause his tinnitus?*

Otosclerosis affects bone in the middle and inner ear, and is therefore quite serious. Beethoven was rather the exception, none the less, in suffering severe deafness and tinnitus. The condition gradually reduces the delicate vibrations caused by in-coming sounds, causing some hearing loss. A sufferer can also become mildly giddy. Fluoridisation of the water supply is thought to reduce the risk of otosclerosis, and the addition of sodium fluoride to the diet can possibly retard its advance. It causes the type of deafness that can be helped greatly with hearing-aids, which can at the same time partly counter the tinnitus which often occurs. An operation is possible, but such surgery carries the risk of causing or magnifying tinnitus, so should not be agreed to lightly.

## Sinusitis

*The racket in my head started six years ago, when I was sixty-three. Am I right in blaming the tablets I was prescribed for sinusitis?*

Probably not. It may be that the infection of the sinus was severe enough to cause toxins in the blood stream and these started the tinnitus. This hardly ever happens in a perfect ear, but anyone in their sixties probably already has some hearing disorder, however slight. Such a disorder can produce tinnitus at any time. A variety of things can trigger tinnitus which is waiting, as it were, to happen. These can range from syringing or a head injury to emotional strain, bereavement or influenza. But you cannot rule out sheer coincidence. Whenever tinnitus occurs it is possible to associate an event, a set of circumstances, or another medical condition with it, but not always accurately.

## Illegal Drugs

*I am a university student and have tried LSD on a few occasions and have smoked a great deal of cannabis. Tinnitus started after a smoking session. Is it true that as I am young the sounds will go away?*

The drugs you mention can have many ill-effects, but tinnitus is not one of them. They are not known to damage the inner ear, though they could just trigger tinnitus in a damaged ear, as so many other things can. Maybe you were listening to very

loud music around the time you took drugs. Amplified sounds
in discos and concerts can certainly bring about the condition. Your age could mean that the sounds will lessen or
disappear, but there is not much comfort to be drawn from
the statistics. A twenty-year-old's tinnitus usually remains
for life. In a minority of cases it also gets worse. Young
people commonly play down the risks to their health, and
exposure to dangerously loud music is one of them.

## A Sound That Can Go

*An ear specialist inserted grommets in both my ears, when
he diagnosed obstruction of the Eustachian tubes, and this
relieved the congestion, but a hissing sound remains. Is
there anything to be done about this?*

Blockage of the tubes reduces hearing, causing a person to
notice more clearly the small amount of tinnitus which can
usually be heard in a quiet environment, if one listens intently
for it. When the blockage is cleared, normal hearing increases
and the hissing disappears. It can, however, remain, as you
have discovered. What you are experiencing should not be
regarded as a threat. Try to ignore it, as thinking about it could
give it a longer lease of life.

## Folk 'Remedies'

*In the past people had great faith in herbal and other
remedies, under the general heading of folk medicine. Is
there anything for tinnitus?*

Books on herbal medicine make many mentions of tinnitus
and suggest 'natural' ways to relieve it. They make similar
claims for many other conditions, of course, and there is
hardly a plant in the garden that is not reputedly a source of
better health. It is understandable that previous generations,
without the range of pharmaceutical products or surgical

methods we have today, turned to the most accessible products of nature to heal themselves. Do not dismiss all of these medicines, some of whose natural properties have been copied in the production of drugs, but unfortunately there is no evidence that the one so-called 'natural' preparation for tinnitus has proved to be an effective treatment.

## A Car Crash Started It

*My back and neck were injured in a road accident, when a vehicle stopped abruptly in front of my car. In hospital a high-pitched noise entered my head—it might have started in the crash, but I was in a state of some shock and may not have noticed it. The sound has not gone, and is temporarily worse if I quickly move my neck or shoulders.*

It seems as if you sustained a whiplash injury. In such cases there are usually no broken bones, but damage to tendons, muscles, nerves or joints. Tinnitus, if it follows at all, can be immediate or after a delay of weeks or months. It usually persists. Injury to the muscles of the neck is known to cause tension in the muscles in and around the ear, and this is thought to be linked to tinnitus. Skilled physiotherapy applied to the neck can bring consequential relief to the tinnitus.

## Hums

*Can the loud hum I hear be tinnitus, or am I particularly sensitive to low frequency environmental noise?*

Tinnitus can be heard as a hum, and can be very loud, while remaining low-pitched. Where the sound has an external source, people have variously blamed underground gas pipes, power-stations and overhead cables. The question is being studied seriously, and the Government has set up an inquiry with the help of the Building Research Establishment. Once the external sources of the sounds have been identified it may be possible to discover if they can cause tinnitus, as well as some people mistaking them for it.

## My Prostate Fear

*I have severe tinnitus, which has badly affected my life. I am willing to try experimental drugs, but am afraid to do so as all strong pharmaceutical preparations have the potential to enlarge the prostate, and I have no wish to add to my problems.*

Your fear is probably groundless, although common enough. Very few drugs cause this. If you have the chance to take part in any proper trials of anti-tinnitus drugs, therefore, please weigh the opportunity on its merits and forget about prostatic enlargement.

## On the Phone

*My tinnitus gets worse when I am on the phone. Because of deafness I have to listen with an ear in which I wear a hearing-aid. Could the pressure of the phone make my noises worse?*

The concentration needed to use the phone can draw attention to tinnitus and make it seem louder. The sound from the phone, which can actually be louder than most speech heard face-to-face, can also aggravate tinnitus. If the phone is held tightly to an ear wearing an aid there can be discomfort, making the tinnitus less easy to bear. You could seek advice on using the phone with a hearing-aid from your nearest hospital-based hearing therapist.

## Nervous Breakdowns

*Nearly thirty years ago I had a mental breakdown, for which I received electrical treatment. Ten years later, at the age of sixty-three, I had a similar illness, and my tinnitus started at the same time.*

Nervous illness itself does not cause tinnitus. Stress, which you may have experienced, certainly can, but usually if there is already some hearing disorder. Such a disorder can come on very slowly, and a person may not know about it until tinnitus starts.

## Coming off Drugs

*I had been taking drugs for depression and insomnia for a long time. When I suddenly came off them tinnitus started in both ears.*

Head noises can start if you stop taking such drugs too quickly. It is always necessary to withdraw from them gradually under supervision. If the tinnitus persists there is usually another cause.

## Unproven, but Harmless

*Would reflexology make my head quieter? I keep reading about it.*

It does have many devotees, but as far as tinnitus is concerned its value remains unproven. Like so many alternative treatments it is harmless, but be prepared to be disappointed.

## But Can it Help Tinnitus?

*I am told that chiropractic can be good for a whole range of physical problems, and can be better than osteopathy. Can it do anything for tinnitus?*

Chiropractic now has official recognition as a proper manipulative therapy. It differs from osteopathy by largely concentrating on the spine and relies greatly on 'high velocity' movements of the body during treatment. It is, however, closely related to osteopathy. It is generally quite harmless, but as rapid and sharp manipulation is widely practised it is prudent to make sure that you are using the services of a properly qualified person. Some chiropractors make claims about relieving tinnitus but there are as yet no convincing statistics in its favour. There have been bits of research undertaken involving a number of tinnitus sufferers but the relief reported by a number of them cannot be scientifically attributed to the treatment they received, as other possible factors have not been thoroughly excluded. However, any course of treatment which makes a patient feel better tends to make him more capable of coping with his tinnitus, which could well seem to diminish. Chiropractic should not, therefore, be dismissed.

### Why is my Tinnitus Better in a Car?

*When I am driving a car or travelling as a passenger my tinnitus seems to reduce and I can hear the radio and other people better. Does this tell me anything about my tinnitus, which I have had (moderately) for twenty years?*

It does not reveal much about your tinnitus but it underlines a useful bit of information regarding hearing for people with tinnitus. A car is, of course, a very small room on wheels and the interior does not have many hard surfaces which make listening difficult for many deaf people. It therefore constitutes, for some people, the ideal environment for hearing. Because you can hear more clearly your tinnitus seems to reduce. If you are driving, the mental and physical effort required also distracts you from the usual level of perception of the noises in your head. It is not possible to replicate the conditions of the car interior in many other places, but the car should remind you that hearing can in part depend on the size of a room and the choice of floor coverings and height of ceiling, etc.

## Am I Likely to Get Ménière's Disease?

*I understand that Ménière's disease and tinnitus are closely linked. As I have had a mixture of noises in my head for eight years and am now thirty-one, am I likely to get Ménière's?*

Statistically you are not likely to experience it, whatever the cause of your tinnitus. Though largely controlled by drugs, Ménière's is a serious medical condition, but it is quite rare compared with tinnitus. It is true that people who have it commonly have tinnitus as a result, but the reverse does not happen.

# 5   Alternative Therapies

## HYPNOTISM

The business of one person putting another into a trance has a special place on the fringe of medicine. With one foot in, or close to, accepted medicine and the other on the stage of light entertainment, there is no other healing practice attracting simultaneously so much keen support and utter condemnation and incredulity. Can it make you better in one context and entertain and amuse you in another? This very diversity of its use is enough to put people off. For them, seeing volunteers doing silly things on the public stage because a hypnotist has told them to behave that way is proof that it has as much reality as a conjuror sawing a lady in two. And if that is the case, what is it doing alongside conventional medicine?

Anyone with tinnitus may, understandably, have a less dismissive opinion. After all, we are told that head noises are more to do with the brain than the ears, and doesn't hypnosis somehow control, or at least influence, the brain? Tinnitus, therefore, has made a few recruits to the army of firm believers—and hopers—marshalled behind hypnotism in its ceaseless fight against the sceptics. Clinical psychologists, some of whom deal with the most distressed sufferers, generally see some value in it, but have to advise against the wilder expectations of anyone hoping for a cure from it.

The keenest advocates of hypnotherapy among professional tinnitus carers point out that noises in the head can require a great deal of psychological adjustment. At the same time, hypnosis allows access to unconscious processes. It is an altered state of consciousness, with changes in memory, mood, perception and sensation. Surely, then, there is something here for treating tinnitus? The answer is a qualified yes. It is nothing like the magic wand of so many hopes, but it is a useful aid in helping people to come to terms with their condition. And sufferers reading this should not sigh 'it's just another way of telling you to learn to live with it' before looking elsewhere for relief. There could be something here for them.

Tinnitus can raise a range of fears and negative attitudes. There can be almost constant worry, for instance, about one's loss of a comfortable social role. This can be just about anything, from not being able to go with friends to a noisy pub to losing reading concentration and a feared consequent inability to keep up with intellectual peers. To counteract these real threats, positive action is required in many directions. Time-consuming hobbies or routine patterns of living may have to be abandoned or adjusted to find the time for medical care. Limitations on quality of life, such as having to miss live concerts, will be a big problem for some. For others, fear of tinnitus and the belief that it will get worse with age may have to be overcome. In all these tasks, a clinical psychologist or counsellor can offer a range of advice and therapies once an individual's case has been properly and uniquely assessed. Often the opportunity to alter the state of consciousness of the patient while the healing attempt is made is a priceless help, and hypnosis can sometimes clear the way to achieving it. It should be looked on as a special adjunct to therapy, making easier the process or psychological environment in which the changes will, if at all, take place.

While wishing to play down the hype and public excitement surrounding the stage hypnotist, hypnotherapists, who are lamentably few in number, none the less want to demonstrate their worth in the quest for good health. They point out that hypnosis is a state of mind in which suggestions involving opinions and actions are more likely to be accepted. A hypnotised person is likely to replace sensory experience with powerful mental imagery, as well as finding it is easier to concentrate thoughts on a narrow subject. He is also likely to be willing to link himself with a form of substitute reality. Such imagined reality can be brought forward by the patient or suggested by the hypnotherapist. There can, for instance, be a suggestion to think about happier, tinnitus-free times. It can also be helpful to talk the person into accepting a generally stronger self-image, to cope better with tinnitus throughout the day.

Hypnosis is used increasingly in the treatment of many medical conditions, always with the warning not to expect too much from it by itself and that it is no magic metaphorical bullet to kill a disease or a symptom. Tinnitus was not the first medical condition to suggest itself as likely to benefit from trance-based treatment, but the two subjects have established what is sure to be a permanent link. And does it really work—or are respectable hypnotherapists, in their own fashion, just as likely to mislead as a hypnotist bent on winning over audiences on TV? There is now no doubt that it can help. The lack of a great number of successful case histories may have more to do with the scant amount of resources available in public medicine than with any inherent weakness in the therapy.

There is also evidence that tinnitus patients are more difficult to hypnotise than the rest of the population. If that is so, it is yet another statistical complicating factor in finding out what hypnosis really is and why some people can enter a trance more easily than others. Is a proneness to fantasy a help? Is there such a thing as human magnetism between two minds? Greater use of hypnosis to beat tinnitus will not need to wait on the solution of these riddles, no more than one has to understand electricity before fixing a plug to a lamp and illuminating a room.

Though unable to stop the noises themselves, hypnosis can be applied directly to alleviate tinnitus-related complaints, including stress, anxiety and sleeplessness. In a number of tinnitus clinics it has, among other things, been used to enable patients to return to coping strategies in which they had lost faith.


## THE TOMATIS METHOD

Head sounds can be an occupational hazard for executives who worry too much about their stressful work, according to one of the latest theories. Innovative treatment consists of listening to music from which the low frequencies have been filtered out. Gregorian Chant is also sometimes used.

The treatment is known as the Tomatis Method, named after Professor Alfred Tomatis of Paris, and is practised in many countries. With singing and speech problems also treated, the organisation claims the late Maria Callas and the actor Gerard Depardieu among its cured patients.

The professor reminds tinnitus patients that one of the many functions of the middle ear is the ability to select what one wants to hear or not. It is possible to listen to only one instrument in an orchestra, and more or less shut off the rest. Similarly in a noisy environment, most people can select one voice or other sound to listen to. Often with age or hearing disorders, people are unable to do this, and are 'invaded by parasitic external sounds'. A fully functioning ear not only cuts off external sounds but the inner sounds of the body as well. These sounds are caused by such things as liquid movement, blood circulation, heartbeat, circulation of the blood, breathing, chewing and molecule movement.

Tomatis claims that some tinnitus appears when the two muscles in the middle ear become tired or damaged, causing a person to hear his own inner sounds. When this happens there is a drop in normal, high frequency hearing. In his words:

This drop is relatively common among people affected by noise trauma such as those in the military, hunters, factory workers or older opera singers. In the elderly, it is generally attributed to the normal ageing process but it is most unusual for adults in their mid-thirties or forties who were never exposed to loud noise or have no family history of hearing loss. However, there is also a striking number of professionals in high-pressure jobs who have this specific listening profile—also called Executive Ear.

It is no coincidence that tinnitus is often related to high blood pressure associated with stress. Listening can also be affected by overwork and continuous pressure. Attention span starts to fluctuate, one becomes fidgety and distracted during meetings, mood swings are more drastic and decisions are made impulsively. The levels of energy start to drop, but one is too busy to pay attention to it. Listening becomes more and more selective, narrow, rigid and tiring. Some people may even start to have a nervous breakdown and suffer from depression.

The use of high frequency music will, it is claimed, enable the ear to 'recharge itself', release many inner tensions and reduce tinnitus.

A machine called the Electronic Ear is used in Tomatis's clinics to enable patients to hear the filtered music, in a number of sessions. The hearing is monitored to measure improvements and reductions in tinnitus are noted.

The Tomatis Method includes a close study of a person's skills and her impairment as well as behavioural and social traits. This is justified on the grounds that as listening cannot be seen, it is necessary to pay attention to a person's total state of fitness and shortcomings, to search for clues to the tinnitus or other debilitating condition. A potential patient is invited to complete a checklist of her own skills or lack of them. Those which seem to apply directly to a tinnitus sufferer include confusion of similar sounding words and hyper-sensitivity to sounds. Apart from its diagnostic value, such preliminary self-examination could be useful in making people acknowledge their hearing and tinnitus difficulties and more readily accept that something should be done by way of positive action.

There have been instances of reported relief among people with tinnitus, but general claims are on the basis of fairly flimsy statistics to date. The treatment is at best a continuing and promising experiment. Deafness accompanying tinnitus is usually of the high frequency type, and many tinnitus sounds can be matched to frequencies. (A musician will, for instance, talk about his single noise as A above middle C or perhaps an F sharp an octave above the treble stave.)

As so many people in the musical world experience tinnitus—from students at the music colleges to instrumentalists exposed to a life-time of sounds in such places as the orchestra pits of the theatre and opera house—the special attention being given to the problem is to be welcomed. 'Musicians and singers who are experiencing problems with their performance will receive treatment designed to open up their hearing in order to perceive the full range of frequencies', says Tomatis. 'The voice produces only what the ear can hear. The problem is in the hearing of the singer or musician. Treatment opens up their ears to all frequencies.'

In cases where there is damage to the inner ear, it is difficult to see how music, however filtered and selected, can be a restorative remedy. But as tinnitus probably has numerous causes, some as yet unknown or not fully understood, there could well be a minority of sufferers who would find their condition and this treatment ideally matched.

## ACUPUNCTURE

The ancient wisdom of the East asserts it has its own recipe for relief of the world-wide condition. It offers, as a supplement to modern management of tinnitus, a treatment whose credentials are found in the traditional medicine of China which dates back thousands of years.

To the less informed westerner, acupuncture is all to do with surgical operations being conducted without pain and with a few pricks of a needle supposedly replacing the usual anaesthetics. Such stories of Chinese practices in hospitals become exaggerated travelling around the world and tend to take on an aura of near-miracle. The actual picture is less clear-cut, with Chinese medical people ready to admit that acupuncture is best seen as something of value alongside 'modern' medicine and not as a replacement for it. Its value in tinnitus treatment becomes acceptable if one agrees a fairly basic (though still scientifically unproven) line of reasoning. Putting needles into the correct parts of the body certainly reduces or abolishes pain and, in the case of operations, prevents it. Interestingly, very loud created sounds are experienced as pain by the unfortunate hearer. Could not, then, acupuncture prove to be an antidote for tinnitus levels well below the pain-inducing threshold?

It is unlikely that anyone, with or without tinnitus, has been experimentally subjected to sound-made pain just to see if the use of needles would reduce or cancel it. Yet there is evidence both in China and elsewhere that tinnitus, at different levels of intensity, can partly yield.

It is sobering to note that practitioners list numerous conditions from allergies to vertigo as promising candidates for their work. Tinnitus sits alphabetically between Thyroid and Tonsillitis and, to the sceptic, prompts the question of whether it is there with little more than hope to sustain it and included just to prop up the catholicity of the claims. As in many other forms of treatment, do not let mere doubt turn you off. There are many genuine-sounding testimonials to tinnitus relief, though it is freely admitted that it does not work for everyone.

In its defence, it must be said that the closer one looks at acupuncture, its origins and long development, the stronger the inclination is to accept it as a path worth exploring. Acupuncture goes back some 3,000 years, roughly when a civilisation geographically closer to the West cut holes in the head to let the evil spirits of tinnitus escape. On the face of it, therefore, the East was, at least at that stage of human malady and treatment, better equipped to treat sufferers. It has remained part of traditional medicine which includes the use of herbs, exercise, massage and diet. It claims to have a unique understanding of the human body. Fine needles are used to stimulate invisible lines of energy running beneath the surface of the skin. A little less certain is the claim that the puncturing of the skin changes the energy balance of the body, thus helping to restore health. Sometimes herbs are burned—known as moxibustion—as a supplement. There is a theory that Stone Age people used sharp bone to scrape the skin or lance boils and to stimulate the body. By accident they found that such points seemed to lie in definite pathways, and the sensation from the needle passed along these lines and had a therapeutic effect on the body. Later in history, knowledge of basic anatomy helped to form the current theories of channels of energy.

But as tinnitus is really a symptom and not a disease in itself, can it find a place in such treatment? As something else is causing it, would it not be necessary first to find that 'something else' and then see if acupuncture could be of use? Such doubts can probably be dispelled by the treatment's 'whole person' approach. Western doctors look for a specific cause or agent of a disease and control or destroy it with drugs or surgery. Chinese medicine also looks at the disease but takes into account the habits and physical and emotional characteristics of the patient and attempts to measure and chart what acupuncturists call patterns of disharmony that have arisen. Good health, it is concluded, is a state of total harmony involving the physical, emotional and spiritual aspects of the person. In many cases the symptoms of a complaint, however severe, are not important. If that is true, tinnitus (in its status as a symptom) also loses importance and could eventually disappear or recede as merely a bit player in the total drama being played inside the body of the sufferer.

The healthy internal balance of the body and the flow of vital energy can be upset by many things, from stress, worry, fear and grief to dependence on alcohol, accidents, falls and hereditary factors. Interestingly this is reflected in the many conditions or events that tinnitus patients often claim as causes or triggers of the head noises, though this is not enough in itself to prove the remedial value of acupuncture for them.

Anyone taking their tinnitus to a practitioner is likely to be treated seriously. To reveal a pattern of disharmony, questions and observations will seek to build up a picture of lifestyle, emotional state, diet, approach to work, etc. Treatment can be combined with western drug therapy, where, for instance, it has been prescribed for tinnitus-related Ménière's disease, or for conditions not associated with head sounds. Treatment for tinnitus is usually once a week or fortnight.

The strongest clinical evidence in favour of this special branch of medicine shows that it can definitely relieve muscle tension in the neck and head. Such tension can cause or aggravate tinnitus. Does this also support the central theory of acupuncture, i.e. that the energy of the body (known as Qi, pronounced 'chee') keeps the blood circulating, warms the body and fights disease? Qi, it is believed, flows through a network extending from the foot to the top of the head, with twelve channels each connected to an internal organ. If this is so, and there has been scant evidence to the contrary, it is unlikely that the ear and its connections to the brain have been somehow omitted from the detailed scheme. And if they are included, is it not possible that some forms of tinnitus are symptoms of this life-supporting flow of energy? Does this ancient form of medicine hold the key to the timeless and baffling mystery of tinnitus?

## SHIATSU

Not far removed from acupuncture, but with its own advocates who claim it is helpful in managing and relieving tinnitus, is

the Japanese form of healing known as Shiatsu. It is sometimes known as acupressure and consists of pressure being
applied to the points and energy lines of the body identified in
acupuncture. The practitioner may use thumbs and fingers,
elbows, knees and feet to stimulate blood circulation and the
flow of lymphatic fluid. Tense muscles are soothed and feelings of calmness and well-being are widely reported. No one
claims it can cure tinnitus, but there is strong evidence that it
can reduce the familiar consequences of it, like sleeplessness, anxiety and depression—all of which can be worse to
bear than the sounds themselves. Where better circulation of
the blood results, some people with pulsating tinnitus have
found marked relief.

Practitioners of Shiatsu like to distinguish it from acupuncture, while acknowledging a common origin. They also
point out, accurately, that it is much older than many more
familiar western therapies, like physiotherapy, and employs
a profounder understanding of the complete body and its
workings. Shiatsu attempts to affect the physical, emotional,
psychological and spiritual facets of a personality. Advice is
sometimes given on diet, exercise and lifestyle, and the
ultimate goal is enhanced self-confidence and peace of
mind, as well as a tangible improvement in health. Confidence and mental stability can be seriously lacking in
people feeling battered by their tinnitus. Without over-
stating its potential or making miracle-like claims for itself,
Shiatsu offers an inviting prospectus. It is, however, strictly
a complementary therapy and should not replace any traditional treatment.


## CRANIO-SACRAL MASSAGE

Accidentally hit your hand with a hammer and the almost
instant reaction is to give it a hard rub to take away or lessen
the pain. An injured footballer or a young child knocking a
knee when falling over may also resort to the same type of
self-administered treatment. Why not, then, rub the head to

stop or reduce internal sounds? The idea has not been totally dismissed as worthless. Rubbing away tinnitus is a simplified way of describing what some osteopaths practise on patients.

The brain and inner ear are the source of tinnitus, and keep their awesome secrets encased in the skull, which provides such wonderful basic protection for them throughout life.

Could it be that the strains and tensions of the head play a part in a person's perception of tinnitus? If so, could not manipulation of the head bring relief, just as relaxation in general is the sole means of relief for so many sufferers? A group of people who think it can are cranial osteopaths, who concentrate their skills on the head. The treatment involved is quite uncomplicated, fairly easily obtained and already has its keen supporters among those who have received it. The osteopath applies gentle but firm finger-tip pressure gradually over the whole of the head and face, usually in treatment lasting less than an hour. The treatment usually needs to be repeated but not for many sessions.

A few patients have reported that their sounds have completely gone and a larger number swear that the relief they have enjoyed has been greater than that from any other kind of treatment.

Similar claims are made for a closely related practice, cranio-sacral therapy, whose advocates are rather more specific in what they say should be done. With tinnitus patients they say there is often a tightness in the temporal bone, which contains the middle ear. By gently manipulating the bone until it has gained its natural rhythm it is possible to reduce tinnitus. The bone tightness can have causes varying from long-term stress to a sharp shock. The tinnitus itself exacerbates the stress, thus creating a circle of cause and effect which needs to be broken.

There is a growing belief that cranio-sacral therapy is the most direct way of releasing resistances in bones, tissues and fluids in the head. In most cases it is likely that the internal tensions are not making the noises, just making them worse. This form of therapy, none the less, may be the best treatment in a limited number of cases. Anything that produces harmless relaxation is worth a try.


## CRANIOFACIAL THERAPY

The human body may be a wonderful intricate machine, with many parts finely dependent on each other, but who would guess that the jaw could be linked to nasty sounds? We know it moves every time we open our mouths to eat or speak, but implicated in tinnitus . . .?

Temperomandibular disorder or TMJ is a distressing, complex and poorly understood condition involving the head, neck and jaw. For reasons unknown, most sufferers are women. Trouble in the jaw, the muscles around it or in the 'bite' results in pain and dysfunction capable of lasting a very long time. Surveys have shown that one person in eight is affected by some kind of jaw pain. TMJ sufferers often also complain of tinnitus, as well as variously chronic headaches, earaches with no infection, dizziness and facial or jaw pain.

The disorder can be caused by imbalance in the jaw/skull relationship following injury in sport or a car crash, whip-lash injury which damages the jaw, clenching or grinding the teeth, misaligned teeth or prolonged poor nutrition which affects muscles in the jaw mechanism.

The fact that most sufferers are women affects the manner in which TMJ is treated. Patients are often wrongly sent to gynaecologists, neurologists, orthopaedic specialists, and finally to psychiatrists. The severe pain is sometimes dismissed as psychosomatic in origin, with antidepressants being prescribed, or the problem is allied to hormonal imbalance. After misdiagnoses, false starts and wrong referrals, patients of both sexes remain in pain and may be bewildered and emotionally distressed. The earlier the disorder is properly diagnosed and treatment started, the sooner a patient can expect a return to health and a reduction or abolition of any tinnitus.

Treatment for craniofacial pain and TMJ disorder has been widely available in America for many years, with many experienced practitioners in the field. In Britain there are few practices totally dedicated to it. One Harley Street clinic alleviates pain in the muscles around the face by using ultra low frequency transcutaneous electrical neural stimulations (TENS) and cranio-sacral therapy to relax the muscles. Later, a splint of clear acrylic is made to cover the lower teeth and hold the jaw in proper alignment. Relaxation and stress relief, osteopathic manipulation and nutritional advice are also beneficial. The whole treatment package does not involve surgery or drugs and always takes place on an out-patient basis. Most patients need to be seen every few weeks and healing can be expected in six to nine months.

The common phenomenon of 'clicking' jaw, with the joints not quite working properly, but not producing pain, can also mean trouble for a tinnitus sufferer. A hearing-aid or masker can feel uncomfortable as the jaw moves. This can be avoided either by wearing a very light ear mould with the traditional behind-the-ear instrument or an instrument which rests deep in the ear and avoids the 'clicking' trouble spot.

# 6    Living with Tinnitus

As tinnitus is a symptom of something else, not strictly an illness or disease in itself, any discussion of its consequences presents the strange exercise of considering symptoms of a symptom. To that can be added what can be termed the chicken-or-egg dimension, with debate over whether tinnitus causes or worsens another condition, or vice versa. The diagnostic dilemma and the question of treatment are typically encountered on the subject of stress.

Not everyone with tinnitus—even in its worst form—suffers stress or, in its excess form, distress. To those who experience it, however, it appears a self-perpetuating continuum of head noises; a life of tinnitus accompanied by relaxation being for them more of a desperate hope than an attainable goal. Moreover, stress seems to weaken the sufferer's resolve and in turn makes the tinnitus worse. It all makes yet another circle of cause-and-effect needing to be broken.

The subject has opened up a rather heated debate among some sufferers and those who care for them in the healing professions. Therapists say that stress may be the most important treatable facet of the general tinnitus condition. Until a person has learned to calm down and remain calm, tinnitus cannot be further managed or, occasionally, abolished. The counter-argument among some sufferers frustrated by years of failure is that it is a wasteful diversion to concentrate on relieving the stress, which would soon go if the head noises were removed or significantly lessened.

It is not at this stage necessary to take sides in the debate, at least before examining the nature of stress and its importance in so many lives. First, a few basic facts.

Stress does not necessarily cause tinnitus, any more than tinnitus necessarily brings about stress, though they can be closely linked. Stress is not like a deadly virus waiting to attack anyone, but springs from the interaction between what happens and a person's perception of what is happening. Factors that create stress (stressors) and play havoc with the balance between mind and body are present in everybody. Tinnitus is, without doubt, an identifiable stressor, but varies from person to person in how it can affect the handling of the symptom. As one specialist put it, some patients regard themselves as suffering tinnitus while others say they are experiencing it. The 'sufferers' take longer to adjust, even with expert therapy, while the 'experiencers' are able to cope better and lead lives closer to the norm.

## RELAXATION

The surest way to move from suffering to coping is learning to relax. In its most thorough form this does not mean dropping into an easy chair or going to bed. Unless sleep quickly follows, a person seeking relaxation this way may well concentrate more than ever on the tinnitus and this would bring more stress—not so much breaking the circle as drawing it more indelibly. And even if sleep does happen, temporary oblivion is no cure. Relaxation can be learned from therapists on a one-to-one basis or is more cheaply obtained in such places as adult education classes. Meditation, possibly learned at home with the aid of a text book, can mean finding something other than tinnitus to focus on successfully.

If untreated, stress can lead to physical tension, which can cause real pain. Often this is brought about by a build-up of acid in the muscles. Massage can be recommended for dealing with such pain and thus reducing the tension and possibly the original stress.

With so many recipes for stress relief on offer, it is a matter of trying more than one before making a choice, or choices, as a combination is sometimes best of all. Complementary medicines are harmless and gentle, even if they can bring disappointment for some.

The popularity of home entertainment and recorded sound has led to the fastest growing means of reducing stress among tinnitus sufferers. The relaxing properties of music are as old as the art form itself, and the choice and quality of recorded sound reasonably available to all have no doubt enabled people to avoid stress, without their knowing it. It was only a matter of time, therefore, before pleasant and high quality recordings were consciously employed to diminish stress. The result has been the marketing of a whole crop of tapes designed for that purpose.

Stress has mainly the same characteristics whatever its cause. Consequently many tapes have attempted, with some success, to offer a blanket remedy to cover all examples of it. Some have a soft voice calmly recommending simple relaxation techniques, others have a semi-hypnotic effect or rely on natural sounds like rainfall or the breaking of waves, with or without music. The choice of music can pose a problem. The commercial music industry has profitably marketed what they say is relaxing music almost as a genre in itself, often consisting of strings playing the most predictable and undemanding of scores. It has become known as 'easy listening' and there is clearly a market for it. The makers of some relaxation tapes have erred in thinking that everyone has the same tastes. Candy floss music can grossly irritate many people, and if they are stressed it is extremely unlikely to appear palatable to them. More stress could follow it! We may one day see a wide range of relaxation tapes which, where music is included, will offer a choice, from Pergolesi to (softly played) pop.

In recent years therapists and people who have tinnitus themselves have turned their hands to making tapes which take into account the special nature of stress caused by head sounds. Tinnitus, after all, is uniquely a constant, conscious condition and reminds a person of the very cause (or one of the causes) of his stress. The result has been a distinct improvement in quality and quantity of what is available. The relaxing sound in some cases more or less matches some of the softer sounds of tinnitus familiar to millions of people and merges gradually into the more acceptable external sounds of nature. Not all tapes are intended to induce sleep, but at least one carries a warning not to play it while driving a car.

Control of stress is a high priority in advice given to head noise sufferers by the British Tinnitus Association. Its world-wide membership has been told there are four types of stress—mental, emotional, physical and behavioural—and there are many simple ways of reducing them. Sufferers are advised:

Pick out a few from the following list each day and you will soon find yourself feeling less tense and more able to cope with the stress and strain of everyday life:

—Walk/sleep/eat more slowly/linger at the table after a meal
—Leave your watch off
—Drive in the slow lane
—Listen to music/soak in the bath/read (one at a time or all together)
—Recall pleasant memories/contact an old friend
—Practise smiling
—Practise assertiveness
—Practise anger control
—Eradicate hostile grimaces
—Refer to yourself less often in conversation
—Verbalise affection to your family
—Notice objects around you, such as trees and flowers
—Alter one of your usual habits or ways of doing things
—Visit a museum, art gallery or park
—Buy a gift for someone you care for

It is also possible to fight tinnitus just by sitting in a chair, says the BTA:

Frequently our emotions and anxieties are reflected in tense muscles, often twisted and hunched, ready to spring into action. We tend to develop habits and postures which can leave us feeling tired, even exhausted. Learn to sit in a relaxed manner for a feeling of calm and confidence. The technique is:

—Do not wear tight clothing, which causes tension
—Sit well back in the chair, with your back well supported
—Move lower legs forward so that the weight of the upper legs rests on the chair
—Roll your knees and thighs outward
—The buttocks should be spreading
—The abdomen should be soft and loose and the stomach should rise and fall easily with breathing
—Drop your shoulders and feel the back of the neck become longer and your head upright
—Don't press elbows into your sides and rest unclenched hands heavily on your thighs
—Balance your head centrally
—Your tongue should be relaxed at the bottom of the mouth
—Lips should be slightly touching. Think of a smile
—If you feel like it close your eyes or focus on something in the room
—Keep your eyes still and imagine them becoming wider
—Imagine your brow becoming higher, with a smoothness coming over the scalp and down the back of the neck
—Let your body sink into the chair and imagine a feeling of peace

## AVOIDING THE WORST MOMENTS

As with most conditions, tinnitus has its peaks and troughs, good and bad days and fluctuations of intensity. It is a good idea to try to plot and record them in a diary, though it needs a real effort to add regularly to what can be seen as a laborious journal of a loathsome and uninvited companion. The reward comes when a pattern of distress emerges which can point the way to relief. It can only be used remedially—and then only for some people—if the tinnitus graph can be related to an equally detailed record of what food and drink was consumed each day and what else happened in the day-to-day life of the sufferer. What exercise was taken, how much time was spent out of doors, what domestic or occupational stresses there were, what pleasant diversions were experienced ... These and other factors need to be weighed in conjunction with increases or reductions in the noises.

About the commonest of all recorded facts to be thrown up by self-observation—so common, in fact, one can say it hardly needs a place in the tinnitus diary, but implants itself firmly in the minds of sufferers—is that the worst tinnitus can be expected on waking. For millions of people, the most unpleasant moments and minutes are at the start of the day. The tinnitus will also probably reach a high point of intensity and annoyance at the end of the day, and this is explained by the theory that the body is likely to be tired in the late evening and is not up to fighting off, psychologically or physically, the effects of a day of sounds. But why is it even worse, for many, briefly at the start of the day? Surely a body refreshed from a night's sleep should have the best chance of fighting back? Ever resourceful, many feeling greatly challenged by their tinnitus when waking up have found an accessible defensive weapon. A sugary or glucose-laced drink, if their diet allows, quickly brings the excessive sounds to a more acceptable level. The rapid intake of carbohydrate boosts the body's energy and provides, it appears, the extra strength needed to counter some of the tinnitus. Unhappily the remaining tinnitus does not yield to further glucose drinks, but the initial one can see off the additional tinnitus that waking can bring for another twenty-four hours.

But the mystery remains. Why should it happen in the first place? Indeed, why should tinnitus also be much worse for a while after a person has woken from the briefest of sleeps during the day? The common factor is, of course, sleep, not its length nor the time of day when it occurs. Nor, some would say, the quality of the sleep. With no obvious bodily or environmental or social stimulus to which can be attributed the post-sleep worsening of tinnitus, the trail leads to a sufferer's perception of it. And as there is no conscious perception of anything during sleep, the subconscious mind looks like the guilty party.

Set aside for a moment or two what the subconscious mind can or may do to tinnitus, and consider what else it does in sleep. It can, for instance, solve problems that remain insoluble while a person is awake. Struggle with the remainder of that tricky crossword before going to bed and in the morning the answers jump up at you. Try to recall details of a past event at midnight and they can float into your memory the following day before you have thought about breakfast. The great, largely unexplored and uncultivated world of our subconscious mind is not always so benevolent. It can, unbidden, dredge up the worst of thoughts while we sleep and create a horrific world of nightmare as real, for the moment, as anything experienced in the waking, conscious world. Is this not, then, the secret of those enhanced noises heard at the start of the day? Our hidden mind has been given free rein to make what it likes of tinnitus, and parade it through the rest of the mind, in its worst colours, to start the new day. It has to be told to stop misbehaving in such an unseemly fashion.

Earlier in this book the encouraging practice of training the mind to manage tinnitus is explored. A sufferer can condition the workings of the brain so that it is perceived as less threatening and more subject to the will of the person it is affecting. In the most successful cases, the perception of the sounds goes completely, and the one-time sufferers are reintroduced to a world of silence. Some see this treatment as the best hope of relief, pending a breakthrough in drug treatment or surgery. Does the control of the subconscious hold out equal promise?

Anyone who has the spirit and strength to fight their tinnitus throughout the day—or, more correctly, to put it in its place, right at the back of the queue of things awaiting attention—does not have to surrender to it in sleep, when the subconscious is in control.

Strive to implant in your mind the best image of tinnitus, or persuade a suffering friend or relative to do so. Keep trying so that the subconscious mind finally gets the message. The result could even be pleasant dreams about tinnitus. It has been known for the very sounds to be transformed into sumptuous harmonies in sleep. However difficult it is after a taxing day, try to fall asleep with maybe exaggerated but good thoughts about the subordinate nature of head sounds in the context of your whole being and life.

Tell yourself repeatedly that *you* are in charge of events and would like your whole mind, including the subconscious part, to understand that tinnitus must not be given total freedom even when you are asleep. It must not take advantage of your relative helplessness between falling asleep and waking. Constantly wish that the subconscious will occupy those hours bringing to imaginary life the happier experiences and sensations that can put tinnitus to shame.

Each morning, and after a daytime nap, the subconscious will still partly hold sway for a few minutes until the conscious self is fully in control again. That is true even for those who can spring out of bed or an armchair and appear to be properly awake in an instant. But it can be gently taught to be a servant and not a master. The rich reward, for some people, is a marked reduction in that dawn chorus in which the sounds are anything but birdsong.

## CAN DIET MAKE A DIFFERENCE?

The healthy eating or—say the cynics—the food faddery debate of recent years has reached the subject of tinnitus. As the affluent West gives the impression of spending more time debating the supposed dangers of food than actually preparing and eating it, the torrent of words has spilled over into discussions of what on the menu is good or bad for permanent head noises. The conflicting advice it has all generated has left sufferers either rather confused or convinced that there is, as yet, but slender evidence of any link between what is consumed and what is heard.

With every other person seemingly wanting to excel in understanding the finer points of dietary matters, it had to happen that a large number of people with tinnitus should bring forward their own ideas. Variously they are ready to condemn almost any item of food and drink, from red wine and white cabbage to white sugar and red apples, as causing louder noises in the head. Anyone who took all their advice would have the added problem of malnutrition to confront.

To date there is no scientific evidence that the absence or presence of a particular food or drink can influence head sounds. Sufferers seeking advice from doctors are usually lectured sagely about sensible dieting in the interests of general good health but are not given any list of items to eat or avoid for their tinnitus. An otherwise healthy individual is naturally better able to cope with the strains and stresses imposed by any medical condition. Such general advice is therefore an indirect help in countering the worst effects of tinnitus, but that is as far as it should go. Many remain unconvinced, however.

At any meeting of tinnitus people—indeed, in any conversation between just two—dietary fads will often crop up. Alcohol is frequently cited as a major irritant, with red wine receiving most brickbats. Yet the relaxing effects of alcohol can be an aid to coping with tinnitus. A high-fat diet is also blamed for increased noise in the head, but eating a plate of pastries can be so enjoyable that the eater can better face up to his or her noises!

And what does one make of dietary arguments that change so rapidly? Not long ago the common potato was slammed as a fat-making threat to health. Now it is championed as a fat-free, stable and harmless food. Today the battle lines drawn between butter and margarine are perhaps not as clear-cut as opposing sides in that part of the food industry would have us believe. As the words and allegedly expert counsel fly around them, the tinnitus population is left to pick the wheat from the chaff, as it were. But is there anything of use to be picked?

The most important thing to remember is that food is fuel, no different from a tankful of petrol in a car. It gives us energy and the ability to run the complex machine we call our body from hour to hour. Virtually everyone with tinnitus says it is much worse when they are tired, or feeling worn out. Food is no substitute for sleep, but its absence during waking hours can and does induce physical weakness, which itself makes tinnitus feel louder. The basic lesson is therefore: don't starve yourself. Proper eating can be an ally in keeping some tinnitus at bay. As tinnitus is also usually worse on waking, a sweetened or other high-energy drink first thing in the morning can help. Adequate reserves of energy will give a person the strength to put the noises partly in their place, below the highest levels of consciousness. At the other end of the day, going to bed with an empty fuel tank can produce what used to be called night starvation, unsatisfactory rest and a premature awakening with attendant louder noises.

Amid all the confused messages of the healthy food debate, there is the real danger that anxiety about food can itself seriously add to stress already brought about by tinnitus. In such cases it is not worth the worry.

Meanwhile, some people are ready to read too much into indications that a particular food or drink is bad for tinnitus. If red wine does make anyone feel worse, for instance, it is wrong to condemn all alcoholic drinks. If cheese does the same, other dairy products do not necessarily deserve condemnation. Before drawing lasting conclusions about one's diet, it is essential to approach the subject with method and discipline. Changes in tinnitus and variations in diet should be recorded in detail over some weeks, to see if any pattern emerges. A suspect food or drink should be consumed for at least a week and then abandoned for a similar period. But as tinnitus can fluctuate anyway for no apparent reason, the chance of coincidence has to be taken into account if erroneous conclusions are not to be drawn. Giving hasty credence to a food theory can be quite silly. Giving up tea, coffee, wine, meat and cheese, for example, can mean sacrificing food and drink which may have no adverse effect anyway. The resulting lack of enjoyment found in those items makes life less of a pleasure and tinnitus a bigger burden.

As very little is understood about the causes of tinnitus, considerations of diet must remain on the periphery of the subject, but with a scarcity of knowledge at the centre, it is little wonder that the topic of food and drink should attract such passionate discussion at the edge of it.

## CARE OF THE EARS

'Put nothing smaller than your elbow in your ear' is a priceless piece of advice in do-it-yourself health care. No one follows it entirely, but people who have ignored it include tinnitus sufferers. Putting a finger into the head through those two openings made solely for the entry of sounds can mean putting in permanent head sounds. Inserting objects, however seemingly harmless like cotton cleaning buds on a stick, can have the same life-long effect. Less believably, but just as devastatingly, instruments inserted medically for the removal of wax can also leave tinnitus behind.

Because of its extreme sensitivity, the ear, as everyone finds out, can itch maddeningly, and it requires great self-control not to scratch it as deeply as can be reached. The probing and shaking inside the ear can hasten the changes which usually require the passing of time, disease or accident to come about. Deafness and/or tinnitus can result. The commonest weapons people unsuspectingly use to inflict ear damage are the rolled-up corners of face flannels and cotton buds—the latter sold by chemists who should know better and which some ear specialists say should be banned from sale. The damage left by the vigorous application of flannels and buds is the high price sometimes paid by anyone wrongly thinking that such practices are necessary to clean inside the ear or to stop itching. Wax can safely be removed in most cases by the use of ear-drops bought over the chemist's counter, and chronic irritations can be stopped with a very effective drug on prescription. Both can help to avoid tinnitus and deafness.

Yet more hazardous to a minority of patients is an instrument lying, unsuspected, in doctors' surgeries and hospitals—the familiar syringe. People in many countries tell sad stories of how their tinnitus started as a result of an ear syringing to clear wax. Their evidence forms a dossier of damning criticism of a procedure regularly carried out. And for everyone who has complained there is an unspecified number who have accepted that it must have been an extremely rare accident that happened to them. Anyone innocently responsible for giving a patient tinnitus in this way can also find it upsetting. One case history records how a young doctor broke down and wept when she realised what she had done to a man she was trying to help.

Syringing produces both pressure and noise to a dangerous extent. This was confirmed by a Sheffield audiologist as recently as 1994, after he had found that no satisfactory study had apparently been made up to then of the possible connection between the application of water under pressure in the ear and the commencement of head noises. He studied previously reported cases, conducted experiments on a replica of an ear made of silicone and published some serious news for the tinnitus world. A patient with previous but healed damage in the ear could suffer a perforated ear drum due to the action of the syringe. Tinnitus can also be started by the loud sound the syringe makes, where there was already a hearing disorder, even a slight one. One theory is that the efferent nerves of the cochlea in the inner ear are wrongly stimulated, causing the brain to hear tinnitus or to increase it if it is there already. Further, it is believed such triggering can spring from the psychological discomfort and anxiety a person can experience during the syringing. Most people do not have this trouble when they request this effective way of clearing the ears of wax. Indeed, as wax can be a cause of tinnitus, a syringe can actually stop the sounds in a small number of cases. But the hazards remain. If the syringe is to be used, make sure that it is handled with respect in the surgery. It can often be used rather carelessly by an overworked practice nurse. Before agreeing to it, make sure the doctor is reminded of any history of deafness or tinnitus, which may render you too high a risk for such treatment. It may be necessary to visit a hospital as an out-patient to see how best the wax can be removed and to assess any risk of deafness or tinnitus.

A machine that sucks out wax from the ear is less often used, but can also do great damage. Patients have been known to suffer severe trauma from it and to be left with deafness and loud tinnitus. A middle-aged woman in Hampshire is campaigning to have stricter controls on the use of suction machines introduced, and for patients to be fully warned of what can happen to them. Her constant tinnitus has not diminished since a machine 'sounding like a road drill' was used on her in a private clinic to remove wax. She is also deaf as a result. As with syringes, the best advice is to discuss the method of suction thoroughly with a doctor – preferably not connected with the private clinic where it may be carried out—and consider your vulnerability, especially in the light of any existing deafness or tinnitus. Learn if any other method will do.

## HYPERSENSITIVE EARS

Although deafness is never welcome when it arrives with tinnitus, people with head sounds can sometimes actually wish for part-protection from the sounds of the world around them. They want to escape from the everyday sounds of a door closing, conversation or the clatter of tea cups. Everything appears to be far noisier than it should be. A low-pitched voice becomes a shout and other sounds are suddenly unbearable. Someone with tinnitus cannot even therefore listen to the rest of the world for a comforting diversion from his own racket. The condition is also known to those who are only deaf or with otherwise good hearing, but is a particular worry for the tinnitus population. The trouble springs from what appears to be a physical contradiction: a damaged ear, with its own internal noises and perhaps struggling to hear adequately, finds that it is also over-sensitive. A sufferer wishes strongly that there were fewer sounds coming at him.

The condition is known as hyperacusis—a word which has the distinction of being less well known to the public than that of tinnitus! It is caused when the ear assumes the characteristics of a damaged musical instrument—say a piano which has lost its soft pedal and only produces sounds of such loudness they can be heard only with considerable discomfort. Short of living in total silence, however, the sufferer cannot easily close the piano lid, as it were, and walk away from it.

When someone suddenly winces, covers her ears with her hands and asks for less noise in the room, the problem may be hyperacusis. A good ear can hear sounds over about 20 decibels and up to some 110 without immediate discomfort. An imperfect ear affected by hyperacusis can be expected to lose sounds below about 50 decibels but will not easily tolerate those above 80—the noise of a busy street and above which tinnitus can be caused, as it happens. Such levels can be both distressing and painful. In musical terms, the ear has had its dynamic range reduced.

Hyperacusis can usually be traced to loss of some of the tiny hair cells in the inner ear, especially those picking up high frequency sounds such as a flute, a soft door-bell or the song of a bird. As there are consequently fewer hair cells left in the ear, there is impairment of the intricate system of sorting sounds. This in turn means that too many nerve cells are activated together, thus making the person hear exaggerated sound. Even bad tinnitus and some deafness are not enough to drown or mask the often unbearably loud enhanced sounds. The intake of the extra volume is called recruitment.

As the brain determines the perception of any sound, so too the vital ear–brain link is involved in hyperacusis. In all hearing, thousands of fibres in the auditory nerve carry data about each sound to the hearing part of the brain, the journey taking less than a second. En route the signal is processed, including such actions as extracting and highlighting which sounds need to be noted more than others. What the person suffering from hyperacusis finally hears depends on the accuracy of the swift processing. The subconscious brain can, simultaneously, use stored memory to trigger an unfavourable reaction to a given signal, disturbing the person for no easily apparent reason. Serious tinnitus, where present, can cause stress and anxiety, thus making the enhanced external noises even more horrific.

Anyone with both problems should request separate treatment for hyperacusis, if it is not offered. Where a masker is being worn partly to counter the head sounds, care must be taken to ensure that the wrong external sounds are not amplified, thus making the recruitment of sound worse. Many aids can incorporate a feature to 'clip' amplification at the danger level or to provide automatic control of the volume. Just as important, almost, is the choice of ear moulds worn with the aids. Vents in the moulds can determine the amount of unwanted loudness that can escape before it reaches the hearing mechanism in the head.

There are other means of bringing relief. A small white noise generator in the ear can, under careful supervision, help to desensitise the hearing and often defeat the vulnerability to sounds. In a good hospital or clinic this is combined with therapies to reduce the anxiety common in cases of hyperacusis. When a patient is frightened by what he thinks are the dangers of everyday sounds and the fears produce or add to the trouble, counselling is used to expose the fears and allay them.

## SOUNDS THAT ARE NOT THERE

As if the cacophony of known head sounds were not enough, there are also some which are not formally judged to be tinnitus but which can puzzle or torment anyone hearing them. They are strange mysteries uniquely challenging to audiology and to date defying any solution. Some older people, generally already with tinnitus, can hear almost constant music, which can be a complete performance of a work by an orchestra or instrumental soloist, or a song or chorus. The sequence of notes and words is clearly experienced, quite loudly. The sounds have even been known to take the form of childhood hymns which the person cannot recall otherwise hearing for seventy years or more. Doctors have labelled the phenomenon auditory hallucinations, but have got no further in explaining them.

Although viewed with more surprise than alarm at first, the words and music gradually take on the disruptive power of tinnitus and can cause annoyance and anxiety. Musicians and music lovers suffer from it, but it is by no means confined to them. Occasionally a person can quote words or hum tunes apparently unknown to him before the hallucinations commenced. The ready explanation for all of it is that stored memory has involuntarily decided to release the sounds—including those totally forgotten—to the consciousness, and the hearer is helpless to stop them. The striking normality of it, mirroring ordinary listening, tends to place it outside what is otherwise regarded as tinnitus, and the inclination has been to say it is not the 'real thing'. The vague label of 'hallucinations' is conveniently to hand. The hearing of spoken voices, moreover, can indicate mental illness, and it is correct and important to know that tinnitus, though little understood, is not remotely connected with schizophrenia or psychosis. It seems reasonable, then, to disassociate the phenomenon of songs and music from tinnitus and isolate it for psychiatric investigation. The study of tinnitus people who also have this experience suggests that it cannot always be separated, however. It is possible to hear unsummoned music-making in the head without having any mental instability or disease. With the causes of tinnitus still open to speculation, the possibility must remain that in the processes of the brain, the 'hearing' of phantom music is functionally close to the triggering and perception of tinnitus, and may share inner ear nerve defects and distortions. The fact that the sounds of tinnitus can vary from the buzzing of a bee to a jet engine, or a hymn tune to an operatic chorus may be odd, yet they are in extreme cases aural bed-fellows.

In coping with the musical tinnitus, which does not always stay, relief can be gained by using methods suitable for commoner tinnitus, including hearing-aids, white sound generators as maskers and any form of activity or relaxation which the individual finds, through trial and error, to be suitable.

'I would like to live somewhere with no tinnitus for miles around,' was the comment from a West Country farmer when he visited his GP. It sticks in the doctor's memory as one of the oddest remarks he has heard in years of dealing with tinnitus patients. The farmer is one of a growing number of people who complain about low frequency hums in their heads. The sound is not unlike a well-documented tinnitus sound, but can sometimes recede or disappear if the hearer moves to another area. Environmental factors are blamed for it, with underground pipes and cables under strong suspicion. The theory—taken seriously by the Department of the Environment and being investigated—is that electricity and high-pressure pumping can emit sound waves of such low frequency that they can be heard only by people with ears tuned in to low sounds normally below human hearing. Electro-magnetic fields and radar are also blamed. If the sounds can be heard anywhere, the environmental argument obviously can be disregarded and tinnitus acknowledged. Tinnitus can be heard when the body (particularly the head) is in a certain position, such as lying down or sitting. It is therefore possible, for instance, that a person visiting a town and standing up for hours will experience tinnitus which goes again on returning home and sitting down. If the tinnitus happens to be a low hum he could reach the wrong conclusion that the environment in that town is a threat to him.

In rare cases it is possible to hear someone else's head sounds. It is called objective tinnitus, and can be caused by some physical interference or influence of a nerve, cavity, membrane or blood vessel. It is real tinnitus as it meets the essential criterion of being generated within the person, with no external cause or stimulus.

Also rarely, the cochlea can emit sounds without being stimulated. Microphones placed inside the ear can detect and measure the sounds, which have been named spontaneous otoacoustic emissions (SOAEs). The rarity of these is matched by the unusual fact that it is a tinnitus treatable with drugs. Aspirin has been known to suppress it. (Conversely, aspirin, if taken regularly, is believed to cause other types of tinnitus.)

As head sounds are usually long term, it is reassuring to know that one of them is of extremely short duration. It occurs when a person hears a loud bang like an explosion in the head during sleep. Sometimes the hearer screams with the sudden shock and wakes up frightened. The explanation for this is that it could be a harmless but sudden movement of part of the middle ear which causes exaggerated sound signals to be momentarily transmitted to the brain. A sufferer of this 'exploding head' may find it recurs, but at intervals of up to years. The first time it is it heard it can be so alarming it suggests a painful feeling, but this is thought to be imaginary as pain is not reported regularly.

## ATTITUDES TO TINNITUS

Believe it or not, there are those who actually like their sounds. They have become so accustomed to them they would actually miss having the familiar hisses, rattles or hums. 'I know you will think I'm mad, but I have had my tinnitus since my teens and would rather regret it if we parted company now,' a woman approaching sixty once told a startled local self-help group. It is not known whether anyone else expressed such sentiments. But many present, without saying it, probably had come halfway along the road to actual friendly acceptance of something they hated or feared when it started.

Yet the very idea of friendly tinnitus ... Is it merely a cruel joke for many people, especially those who regard it as the worst thing to have happened to them? Before reaching a conclusion, remember that every experience in life can be viewed in different ways by each individual, and its pleasure or pain reduced or enhanced. Unpleasant neighbours who wake you up with a noisy, late-night party will annoy you more than a nice neighbour doing the same thing once in a while, yet your sleep loss is the same in both instances. It is easy to view the situation as more benign if the culprit is not an objectionable source of the nocturnal noise. Why, then, should not tinnitus, so subjective and personal, be viewed from a different angle instead of, as it were, face on and as public enemy number one?

It takes a wrench of concentration to embrace an objective attitude towards heavily subjective tinnitus. Steel yourself to the task. Unlike most other rackets and dins around us every day, it does not come from anyone else. It comes from neither a nice nor nasty neighbour. It is all yours! It is human to wish—to long for—it to go away. But first ask yourself the question: is it an invader of your living space or just a quirky trespasser? Is it someone in your garden planning a robbery or an eccentric individual claiming squatters' rights by setting up home in a tent under the apple tree? We all live by imagery. Why not employ it to some advantage in the quest for relief? Of course it is not necessary to choose tents and apple trees as aids to reconciliation with your tinnitus. Help yourself to the diversity of thoughts and suggestions on offer in your mind. Pick an analogy to fit you like a bespoke garment. If that fails, try the imaginative tools employed by others (yes, even the tent and the apple tree!). Least of all, do not be embarrassed by what you are doing. It is not silly or strange. The Wizard of Oz soon shrank in size and unpleasantness when someone stood up to him—and the greatest truths are to be found in fiction. It is good psychology to look your tinnitus monster straight in the eyes and tell him you have a much more pacific role for him. He may not yet have the decency and good manners to leave your house completely, but after a while you may find him to be no more of a threat than a household pet. What creature has a fiercer face than a bulldog, yet it won't even bark at strangers if it spends too much time on your lap eating milk chocolates.

Cutting the perception of sounds down to size also has almost another person waiting to help—the subconscious mind. No deep understanding of psychology is required to know that we are openly aware of only a fraction of the things we do throughout the day. Turning a door handle or picking up a book involves tiny parts of the body in movements most people do not understand or consider. The hidden mind knows all about it and handles the complex instructions to limbs and muscles. Likewise our attitudes to tinnitus are shaped by what we are not always conscious of thinking. The subconsciousness in every individual is certain to be influenced by our initial reactions to an unpleasantness and in turn gives an automatic conscious colouring to the subject whenever we think about it. The circle of fear and horror can be broken largely by retraining the subconscious mind to stop siding with tinnitus for a change. You can recruit its happy services in many ways, and there is a choice of literature on this life-enhancing method of finding better health. Briefly, tinnitus must be put in its rightful place, as something that can mar or spoil but not destroy . . . There will always be harmful insects in the garden, but should they stop you enjoying the flowers and lawn? Do blots and spelling errors on an original manuscript lessen the enjoyment of a beautiful poem? The next time the subconscious dredges up bad feelings about tinnitus, try to realise that it is acting under orders—your earlier orders. With patience it can be taught dutifully to bring a happier picture to the surface. Few people can be expected to befriend their tinnitus. It is none the less within a sufferer's grasp to reduce its status as a beatable foe, and thus to lighten or abolish the suffering itself.

It is futile to try to cure a headache by hitting the head against a wall. Nor is that a good way to knock a wall down. If the wall itself is annoying it can be neutralised or even made a source of pleasure by, say, decorating it. Get the subconscious mind at work and give that wall of tinnitus a pleasanter hue.

## DOES FLYING AFFECT TINNITUS?

Whatever those lush advertisements from the airlines tell us about its comfort, flying gives rise to fear, however well disguised, among passengers. The safety statistics, the pleasant ambience and the state-of-the-art technology have never quite calmed everyone's nerves between check-in and safe arrival. A serious medical condition can also put flying out of reach of the sensible. So should tinnitus oblige

you to go by sea or road? Air pressure, after all, changes
greatly thousands of feet up in the sky and passengers' ears
do 'pop'. Could the swift pressure changes affect the
ears to such an extent that tinnitus is either started or
increased?

The conventional wisdom is that flying is not a threat. A
pressurised aircraft cannot affect the inner ear, where the
cause of tinnitus is believed to lie. Anyone afraid that the
noise of the engines will make tinnitus louder can avoid
much of the noise by selecting a seat in front of the wing.
Soft ear-plugs can also help. People with ear-worn masking
devices should wear them during flight. Hearing-aids should
also continue to be used in planes. It is sometimes said that
tinnitus increases on an air voyage, but this can have an
innocent explanation. A blocking of the Eustachian tube can
cause an apparent enhancement of the permanent noises, but
this disappears as soon as the tube is cleared. In very
rare cases the change of pressure is thought to affect the
inner ear, but any adverse change to the tinnitus is also
temporary.

What happens to the middle ear can be alarming and
is largely unavoidable. Perhaps the worst sensation
involves the ear drum. The middle ear contains the vital
tiny bones which conduct all sound to the inner ear. It is
normally filled with air at the same pressure as the
surrounding air. At the start of a flight the pressure in the
plane slowly reduces, but the higher pressure in the ear
simply blows the internal air down the Eustachian tube,
which runs to the back of the nose. As the plane descends
to land, however, the factors are reversed. The air in the
middle ear is lower than that in the plane. As a result, the
Eustachian tube can become obstructed and the small
throat muscles which usually open it may not be up to the
task. The ear drum is pressed inwards and there is a
discomforting sensation. But the condition nearly always
corrects itself as the tube clears. The ear drum is much
stronger than generally imagined and can easily withstand

fairly small changes in pressure, however alarming they can be.

To help air passengers avoid difficulties with the Eustachian tube, the BTA has suggested four rules to follow:

1   Make sure you are awake before the aircraft begins its descent (the initial descent from cruising altitudes may be an hour or so before landing). The Eustachian tube does not open effectively during sleep.
2   Keep swallowing, using a glass of water (or your favourite beverage!) at regular intervals; if necessary every 15 to 30 seconds. If this does not clear the ear, pinch the nose between finger and thumb and gently blow air down it with the mouth closed, but without releasing any air.
3   Avoid flying with a cold. With any infection around the nose and throat, the lining of the Eustachian tube is swollen and blocks more easily. If you are forced to travel with a cold, use nasal decongestant drops or spray on the advice of your doctor. Use the decongestant before and during the flight.
4   If you are worried about your Eustachian function and whether it is normal, it is very easy to check on this by a simple test called impedence audiometry. These tests are available at audiology departments, and quickly measure whether your Eustachian tube is normal, and your middle ear pressure is the same as the surrounding atmosphere.

Whatever practical advice is given and taken, there remains a real psychological problem for people strongly fearful that flying brings a tinnitus risk. They wonder—and worry—if the risk outweighs the convenience and speed of air travel. And if they suffer from depression or anxiety because of their tinnitus, the problem magnifies itself and the worry grows. What is probably intended to be an enjoyable experience, such as a start to a holiday, takes on a nightmarish quality. Some take the firm decision never to fly, and are delighted to find that more leisurely modes of travel bring their own therapeutic compensations.


## THE TINNITUS ALPHABET

A guide to living with tinnitus yet partly banishing it can be found in an A–Z list of advice and basic truths. Occasionally reading it—or better still, committing it to memory—will bring its own rewards.

A   is for ACCEPTANCE. Learn to accept your tinnitus and you are on the way to recovery.

B   is for the BATTLE you will have to fight but you will not be alone. Many people are ready to help you and give you all the information known to date.

C   is for CALMNESS. Stay as calm as you can. Getting agitated about your condition will only make it worse. It is also for CONCENTRATION. Try to concentrate on anything except your tinnitus.

D   is for your DOCTOR. Talk to him about your fears and worries regarding tinnitus. Ask him for a referral to a specialist.

E   is for EXHAUSTION and EXASPERATION. The early months are the worst but it does get better.

F   is for your FAMILY and FRIENDS. They cannot hear your noises and they will find it difficult to understand your mood swings and what you are going through.

G   is for the GOAL that lies ahead. You will beat tinnitus although in the early stages you will find it difficult to believe.

H    is for HELP that you will find in many places, including local self-help groups.

I    is for INTERESTS. If possible, take up an interesting hobby, to help to take your mind off yourself.

J    is for JOY, the inner contentment that will help you overcome tinnitus.

K    is for KNOWLEDGE. Find out all there is to know about tinnitus.

L    is for LIVING. After a while your life will gradually return to normal, after the onset of your condition.

M    is for MASTER. Learn to master your tinnitus— don't be its slave.

N    is for NONSENSE. Do not believe the old wives' tales you will be told.

O    is for OPTIMISM. All round the world research is progressing. One day there will be a breakthrough.

P    is for PERSEVERANCE. If necessary change your way of life, but whatever you decide persevere until you know you have won the battle.

Q    is for QUESTIONS. Ask as many as needed to put your mind at rest. Unanswered questions can be a torment.

R    is for RELAXATION, most important to combat stress caused by tinnitus.

S    is for SLEEP. Insomnia can be cured, even if the tinnitus causing it cannot be, yet.

T   is for TELL. You should tell your family and friends how you feel from time to time. They may not intend to forget about your condition, but they do.

U   is for UNFAIR. You may feel it is unfair that you have tinnitus, but there are worse things in life.

V   is for VOW. You should vow to yourself that you will overcome your problem.

W   is for WALKING. A daily walk brings relief.

X   is for X-RAY. If you are worried that tinnitus is the sign of a serious illness in the head, ask for an X-ray. Rarely is anything found.

Y   is for YOU—the only one who can overcome the difficulty. With a little help you can succeed.

Z   is for ZEAL. You must have the willingness and determination to regain the foot-hold you may have lost in life.

# 7 Legal and Social Issues

## NOISE REGULATIONS IN THE WORKPLACE

As modern living appears to get noisier for all, the source of the loudest and longest exposure to sounds remains the workplace. Though working conditions have improved steadily throughout the twentieth century, the unseen horror which threatens the ears has yet to be exorcised. Tinnitus has a fertile breeding ground in the factory and workshop. It claims victims daily.

Governments have acted to point out the danger of noise and impose obligations on employers and employees to minimise or eradicate the threat. Tinnitus has been acknowledged as an avoidable affliction alongside deafness.

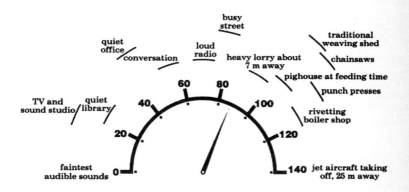

*Some typical levels of sound, measured in decibels. Anything over 80 can cause tinnitus.*

Exposure to 85 decibels is said to be the danger threshold in the Noise at Work Regulations published by the Health and Safety Executive. A sample list of noises above that danger line cites (in ascending order) a heavy lorry about 7 metres away, a traditional weaving shed, a pighouse at feeding time, chainsaws, punch presses, a riveting shop and a jet aircraft taking off, 25 metres away. Repeated exposure to those sounds, and many more, can cause tinnitus, with or without deafness. If ears are already damaged, quite a short exposure can bring permanent sounds.

The Health and Safety Executive has given the following stern warning to the working population: 'You may not notice hearing changes from one day to another, but once the damage is done there is no cure.' It explains how tinnitus can start. Sounds and speech can become muffled, 'a distorted sense of loudness' can be experienced and everyday things like a telephone will be difficult to use. 'You should not have to suffer damage of this sort because of noise at work. It can be prevented by reducing noise level, for example by fitting enclosures and silencers to machines, and using ear-plugs or ear-muffs properly if you have to work in noisy areas. The Noise at Work Regulations say what you and your employer must do. But the danger is only likely to be controlled effectively if you and your employer co-operate to make sure noise levels are assessed and that control measures work properly.'

Earlier enforcement of noise-control laws would have saved generations of workers from serious tinnitus. The changes brought about by the Industrial Revolution rapidly exposed the new class of labour to constant rackets unknown in the rural economy, and the workday sonic pollution continued to ravage its innocent victims through the ensuing centuries. With conversation impossible above the roar of their machines, cotton mill workers in northern England often claimed they were the best lip-readers in Britain. The current regulations represent an enormous advancement in the quest for industrial health, but they are open to the charge of being too little too late. One criticism is that the 85-decibel threshold has been set too high, as tinnitus can be triggered by constant noises in the low-80s.

An employer must have the noise assessed when exposure looks like reaching one of the decibel 'action levels' laid down by the Government. If anyone has to shout or raise their voice to be heard by someone just two metres away or if ears are ringing at the end of a day's work, enquiries should be made to see if the noise has been fully investigated and measured. If a certain action level (taking into account decibels and length of exposure) has been reached, the employer is obliged to say where the noise levels are high and warn about the risks, control the noise, provide employees with ear-muffs or plugs and put up signs showing 'ear protection zones'. For their own part, employees aware of the possibility of tinnitus and wanting to avoid it should follow this advice from the Health and Safety Executive:

1   Use noise control equipment provided. If you work at a machine which is meant to have silencers or enclosures, make sure they are always in place and working properly.
2   Use ear protectors. Wherever there is a serious risk of hearing damage your employer must provide you with ear protectors and you must wear them. In areas where the risk is not so high, your employer has to offer you ear protectors. It is in your interests to use them.
3   Look after your protectors. Learn how to use them. Damaged, dirty protectors won't work properly.
4   Don't ignore faulty equipment. If you find something wrong with noise control equipment, tell someone.
5   If you think there is something wrong with your hearing, see your own doctor or the works medical department.

The advice, and rules, if followed unfailingly, are good enough to save many from tinnitus. Why the duties of employers and employees should be less stringent at 85 decibels than at 90 is, however, not clear, as it is known that head noises can start from exposure to the lower level. Some employers and their organisations have argued that a more stringent application of the regulations would place an inordinate burden on industry, the cost of it being out of proportion to the tenuous and debatable gains. With tinnitus for so long having such a low place in health-care priorities, it is not surprising, yet unfortunate, that consideration of economy may have weighed heavily in setting the danger level at 85 decibels. Up to 90 decibels, for instance, it is not obligatory for an employer to reduce noises by means other than offering ear protectors. Nor is it necessary to mark 'ear protection zones' with notices. And until the 90-decibel level is reached, workers are not compelled to use protectors.

Enforcement of the regulations can be difficult. Road workers using electric drills are often unsupervised and judge wrongly that short bursts of the very loud noise they make can always be tolerated by their ears. Young men, who may think that the risk can be brushed aside in the way they discount that buzz in the ears that sometimes follows a pop concert or a disco have been known to boast that they are strong enough to dispense with ear muffs.

## CLAIMING COMPENSATION

Employers and others can be sued for damages if they can be proved to be responsible for someone's tinnitus, either through exposure to noise or through physical injury. There are many case histories which serve as points of reference for any sufferer who thinks he or she has a case worth pursuing. Most actions are settled out of court, and figures between £5,000 and £15,000 are commonly agreed as damages. There has been at least one agreed settlement of £75,000. In a High Court case, £120,000 was awarded against the Central Electricity Generating Board in favour of a man with a constant shrill whistling in his head. It was claimed the noise was caused by the sounds he was exposed to when visiting power stations. Most of the award, however, related to loss of earnings so no great amount of money was paid for the suffering itself. In some cases where tinnitus has been the only basis of a claim, damages have been greater than in deafness-only settlements. Where deafness has been the chief medical condition, the sum is sometimes increased to take account of tinnitus accompanying it.

Lawyers and judges experienced in industrial injury claims find they have to weigh difficult factors unique to tinnitus before attaching blame and assessing damages. It is known, for instance, that only about one person develops bad tinnitus out of every twenty men and women exposed to identical noisy working conditions. This suggests that the unlucky person may have been predisposed to developing it at the workplace. If he already had some hearing impairment, the employer's claim that the tinnitus would have started anyway in the quietest of environments cannot always be easily dismissed. The coincidence or causal association of deafness and tinnitus is also a complicating factor. Hearing loss can be measured quite accurately, but there is simply not the technology to measure tinnitus. Additionally, tinnitus fluctuates for about a fifth of all sufferers, including many of those claiming damages, or can be intermittent yet very troublesome when it is present. Thus the degree of disability and annoyance can depend largely on what the claimant says it is, and his honesty can be checked only indirectly.

Pursuing a medico-legal claim for tinnitus damages can be as complex—and as expensive—as any comparable civil action. It is realistic to expect evidence regarding the alleged negligence by an employer, the degree of the tinnitus and its overall effect on the victim to be challenged and an attempt to be made to lump the tinnitus element with deafness, if the claimant has both. With the legal costs certain to be high and the outcome rather uncertain, employees are advised to enlist the help of a trade union, whose solicitors will be familiar with the subject. If this is not possible, help can be obtained via the local Citizens' Advice Bureau or from a law firm participating in the legal aid scheme.

Compensation can sometimes be obtained from the Department of Social Security. Tinnitus alone does not qualify for a disablement award, but if there is a 20 per cent or more disability due to industrial deafness, the amount may be increased because of tinnitus.

## TINNITUS AND INCAPACITY BENEFIT

About every twentieth adult with tinnitus finds that it badly affects what researchers classify as 'normal life'. That means that some basic, everyday functions are beyond them—and that often includes following paid employment. Some 200,000 men and women have their 'normal' life troubled. In the next-best category, twice as many adults report that their quality of life—going to the cinema or theatre, for instance—is adversely affected. Many of these find employment increasingly difficult and ultimately impossible. There is thus a huge but uncountable slice of the population incapable of earning a living to support themselves and dependants, because of tinnitus.

In a welfare state one should be able to expect proper financial help for anyone laid low by a condition well known to the medical world but still without a cure or much relief. The reality is soberingly otherwise. As if to complete painting the picture in which official research and health-care neglect are already vividly on the canvas, the state has effectively added parsimony and indifference where individual cash help is concerned. A sufferer unable to work or anxious about how long he can hold down a job needs to be well briefed to face the increasingly hostile environment encountered when seeking social security payments.

Claiming medium or long-term benefits has always been a tricky exercise. Tinnitus cannot be seen or measured by anyone else, so how can it be proved that a claimant is telling the truth when he says he is unable to work? Until 1995 the family doctor was able to certify unfitness for employment, drawing on the patient's case history and the trust established over years of contact in the surgery, as much as the person's stated claim of incapacity. But that has been changed in a radical reform of the whole system of payments. The old invalidity benefit has been replaced by a new incapacity benefit and for anyone with tinnitus the change is more significant than an alteration in name. Claimants are now asked to complete a questionnaire about their ability to carry out specific tasks and work-related activities. The GP is asked to supply details of the patient's medical condition. The Benefits Agency can then arrange for an examination by its own medical staff and, on the basis of the findings, declare that the person is fit to work and refuse benefit payments. It all appears to be a reasonable system, designed in part to act as a counter to bogus claims. Under the surface, however, there are disadvantages for the countless thousands of genuine claimants among tinnitus sufferers. Before the new law was introduced, the Department of Social Security changed its mind and deleted tinnitus from the list of 'functional incapacities'. The nature of the questionnaires used in the new scheme makes it difficult for a claimant with head noises, even severe ones, to score the 15 points needed to qualify for incapacity benefit. A quick examination by a strange doctor will also be less likely to assess the severity and disabling extent of the tinnitus than would a considered assessment by a family doctor. Certainly the filling in of a form and tests such as lifting weights and walking can never reveal the fluctuating nature of tinnitus, which in many cases can make employment impossible on random days. This on-off pattern of incapacity, totally unpredictable, can frustrate even the person with the keenest intentions to find and keep work. Most serious of all, the effect the condition has on concentration and mental alertness will be less sympathetically and accurately assessed in the seemingly harsher new regime of giving financial help to those who find employment impossible.

Tinnitus-burdened claimants need to prepare their case thoroughly. They should discuss the matter with their doctor so that they can at least express their disability in substantive medical terms as well as subjective expressions of the sounds and their effects. Agency officials will need to be told of the unseen, psychological effects and how these relate to an individual. Tinnitus lobbyists who approached the DSS as the legislation was being finally drafted stressed that 'where tinnitus dominates a life, that life can become unbearable, with the consequence that keeping a job becomes increasingly stressful and ultimately impossible'. The Department replied: 'The tinnitus category, which was included in an earlier list of functional incapacities, was dropped following further consultation and evaluation of the all-work test. Though tinnitus can clearly have an effect on capacity for work it is not, in itself, a discrete functional area.'

So Whitehall made up its mind. The medical condition third only to incurable pain and paralysis among the non-fatal challenges to mind and body was pushed further down the list of socio-medical concerns of the Government. In a reform openly acknowledged as a means of economy and a way to root out malingerers, some men and women with this chronic disability will be denied assistance. This is the conclusion to be drawn from a scrutiny of the typical components of the test a claimant is expected to undergo. The qualifying 15 points can be partly scored by not hearing a voice properly in a quiet room (10), not being able to pick up a 5 lb bag of potatoes (8), being unable to take a phone message properly (2) and by being confused in conversation (2). As it is possible to have good hearing despite terrible tinnitus and to be able to do many physical things, tinnitus alone is unlikely to win qualifying recognition.

## THE INVISIBLE WAR WOUND

Of all those who protest at the neglect of tinnitus in Britain, many ex-servicemen and women have the most justification to complain. They have, for the rest of their lives, the invisible wound of tinnitus, which attracts little or no recognition as a disability deserving of financial compensation. Successive governments have declined to acknowledge the plight of many thousands who have this unpleasant reminder of their days in uniform.

There are now generations of former soldiers, sailors and airmen with service stretching back many decades still hoping to obtain a disability pension for a condition that has seriously affected their civilian life. They are drawn from all ranks of the services. For them the basic problem is an unchanging one: how to convince the authorities that constant sounds in the head constitute a totally separate medical condition more burdensome than many of the visible wounds sustained on active service.

It is easy to imagine how the trouble can start for members of the armed services. Loud guns, exploding shells and bombs, noisy aircraft and machinery in confined spaces on board vessels can all prove too much for the delicate mechanism of human hearing to bear. When tinnitus results, it sometimes even resembles the actual sounds that caused it.

One ex-sailor tells how his tinnitus started when his ship was torpedoed in 1942: 'I had to jump from a good height and I can remember going deep into the water, never thinking I was going to surface. I had this ringing in my ears when on a raft for three days before we were rescued.' An Ulster man who was a weapon training instructor during twenty-four years of army service experienced his first 'bumping, banging, ringing and buzzing' in his head in 1955, and had been given no protection for his ears during his noisy duties. Later he was told that his sounds were part of his deafness, and is still wondering 'how they can put two complaints into one category'. Three years' service as a radar operator with a heavy artillery battery in the war-time defence of London gave tinnitus to a woman now living in Crickhowell, Monmouthshire. She is bitter that her permanent sounds have been completely ignored by the pensions authorities. Her feelings are shared by a Market Drayton man. After twenty-two years' service in the Royal Air Force he is 'being driven mad with tinnitus, and feels wronged and let down'. In Paisley a Scottish woman had to give up her career as a secretary, defeated by the constant sounds she traces back clearly to the port of Stromness in the Orkney Islands, where she helped to organise the arrival and departure, in constantly noisy conditions, of huge numbers of soldiers undergoing training for the invasion of France in 1944.

And disappointment awaits many others applying for a war pension. Nearly always there is some hearing loss also, and the applicant is told that his or her tinnitus is regarded as 'part and parcel' of the hearing condition. What is more, there is no pension even for deafness if the hearing disability is measured at less than 20 per cent. Yet it is possible to have serious, permanent tinnitus with little or no deafness. 'What can I do to get them to believe me?' asked a former Royal Artillery man who saw service in North Africa and Italy in the Second World War. 'My deafness is quite slight, and doesn't worry me. Yet my tinnitus is bad, all the time. How can it be dismissed as "part and parcel" of my hearing condition?' His case illustrates what some doctors and lawyers working for ex-service organisations regard as the cruellest injustice endured by people still fighting for their rights. Deafness and tinnitus are quite different from each other. As long as they are lumped together—to save public money, it is thought—justice will remain a casualty of war.

In spite of this, it is not unknown for a pension award to be increased because of tinnitus, so it is worth applying. The claimant has to undergo a medical examination—usually arranged locally—and any hearing loss will be measured. The whole process is a lengthy one, and it is common for a year to elapse before a pension (if any) is granted.

The Government's decision in 1993 to scrap all pensions for new claimants with deafness disability below 20 per cent was a serious blow. Ex-service personnel with little deafness but distracting tinnitus cannot even have the latter recognised as 'part and parcel' of their award if no such compensation can now be gained. It means they are further isolated and barred from benefits. The Department of Social Security argues that the money so saved on deafness pensions is going to pay for upward equalisation of pensions for all ranks in the armed forces. But critics point out that the savings will many times outweigh the cost of making pensions equal for all. Moreover, the arbitrary treatment of deafness as a condition whose benefits can be reduced separately for another purpose, however laudable, lacks fairness. As a consequence of the 20 per cent ruling, the injustice of further exclusion and neglect of the case for tinnitus makes the changes even more deplorable.

Despite all the difficulties, those who think their tinnitus was caused by their time in uniform, even if it came on after returning to civilian life, are well advised to make a claim. Because of what has happened to so many claims in the past, they should half-expect rejection but should be prepared to make an appeal against any negative finding. At any hearing the claimant will usually face a tribunal of medical, service and legal representatives. The atmosphere is friendly and, on the surface, informal. Thorough preparation of the case for a pension is essential, however, as is the ability to ask and answer questions in a procedural framework. Many successful applicants have been glad that they sought the advice of an organisation such as the Royal British Legion beforehand. A good memory—preferably supported by written evidence—can make all the difference. If, for instance, an ex-serviceman cites a particular physical wound as a cause of tinnitus, the description of the battle or incident that caused the wound and the medical record of any ensuing treatment for it, will all become factors to be weighed before a decision is made. The length of any delay between the onset of tinnitus and the date of the pension claim may also have to be explained.

## THE NHS AND TINNITUS

Britain's grand concept of free, cradle-to-grave medical care for all will doubtless always have both admiration and criticism.

The quest for good health, rising standards of living and material expectations are placing growing demands on a service with finite resources and an expanding population to satisfy. The National Health Service, even and universal in its design after the Second World War, presents an uneven and selective national picture today. More GPs in one area, longer waits for surgery in another, dilapidated buildings here, good out-patient services there. In the mixed litany of praise and condemnation it is still rare to hear an allegation that a complete medical condition—and a serious one at that—lies neglected everywhere, receiving a fraction of the attention it deserves. Yet such has been the fate of tinnitus.

As most people fortunately do not have head noises, and have very little knowledge of the subject until perhaps a relative or friend is seen to suffer, there has never been a popular clamour for greater attention to be paid to it by the NHS. And from its onset sufferers are too upset, or passively grateful for the little the NHS does offer them, to protest at the public inadequacies of the treatment available. Yet gaping inadequacies there certainly are, and sufferers can ultimately benefit from being reminded of them.

Today the public is better educated than ever before on medical matters. It is true that the NHS can take credit for some of this wider public knowledge, partly through its active role in telling the nation how to avoid the risk of sickness. There is also a laudable tendency to demystify illnesses and what can be done about them via the family health centre and the hospital. But tinnitus remains an unexplored country, with few signposts to its position on the map of public health. So much so that when anyone hears sounds in the head for the first time it is unlikely that he will relate them instantly to any stored general knowledge of the subject. Indeed, he is not likely to know the word 'tinnitus'. Nor may he instantly recognise it as a medical condition, likely to stay with him for life. A visit to a GP is therefore commonly delayed, and at the surgery disappointment, or worse, may await him. The average GP has no more than a basic understanding of tinnitus, having spent the briefest of time on it during his student days, and despite the statistical certainty that one in ten of his patients will come to him with it at some time. He may check the ears for wax—an occasional and treatable cause—and enquire about any knock or accident that may have brought it on. But if countless complainants are to be believed, the usual final response from the busy GP is the numbing words 'There is nothing to be done—you'll get used to it.' Some people recall how they left the surgery feeling suicidal, when such parting words joined the tinnitus to ring in their ears.

Such a response can be explained and excused if one considers the sad fact that there is little a GP can do, within his own resources. There is no reason for him not to refer the patient to the local hospital for specialist examination and a diagnosis, yet sufferers have sometimes been obliged to change their doctor just to get a hospital referral, after a GP has declined to write the necessary note.

What is on offer at the hospital illustrates vividly how good or bad the NHS can be. The chances are the patient will discover that tinnitus is the Cinderella complaint receiving perfunctory attention in a busy Ear, Nose and Throat environment. Overworked staff will silently regard it as an added trouble sometimes experienced by those with deafness and stubbornly not yielding to treatment. There will be little, if any, attempt to assess and treat the common consequences of tinnitus, such as anxiety, depression and insomnia. At best there will be a hasty suggestion to 'try a masker'—the ear-worn instrument whose own sounds can drown out the tinnitus. There will also be a hearing test to see if there is any accompanying deafness, and that is about all.

Campaigners for better facilities throughout the NHS have
been dismayed to find that the Department of Health has not
even accumulated any central statistics on how many hospitals give a service. Even worse, no minimum standards or
guidelines have been set for hospitals to follow.

While anyone attending a hospital for advice and
treatment has more than an even chance of encountering
poor service, parts of Britain have quite the opposite on
offer. Dundee, Cardiff, London and a number of other
places have hospitals providing a comprehensive range
of facilities, from examination and investigation to the
fitting of maskers and special counselling. An outstand-
ing example of what can be done with adequate resources
and the correct co-ordination of the anti-tinnitus aspects
of audiological medicine can be found at the Nottingham
Tinnitus Clinic. It was set up in 1980—in the early days
of the brief history of serious tinnitus care—and is part of
Nottingham University NHS Hospital. This unit could
well be copied anywhere to the lasting advantage of the
tinnitus population. Each new patient is seen at some
length by a consultant in audiological medicine, who,
after an interview and examination, explains the likely
future course of the condition and possible treatment.
Where appropriate, blood tests and X-rays are suggested.
Displaying a degree of care not even remotely offered in
most towns, the clinic gives the new patient a booklet
which, in a section headed 'Treatment of Cause of
Tinnitus', states: 'Unfortunately, it is still rare to find a
cause that can be corrected leading to abolition of
tinnitus, but a search is always made and appropriate
treatment offered for any such causes when discovered.'

The next section, 'Tinnitus Masking and Retraining',
explains: 'Where there is some hearing loss, retraining
and partial masking are often achieved with a hearing-
aid. If this gives insufficient relief, we may go on to a
trial of two hearing-aids or to give a special device which
generates its own noise, called a tinnitus retrainer, or

both. The tinnitus retrainers we use are usually small in-the-ear devices, but occasionally are more like behind-the-ear hearing-aids.' It adds: 'In other cases, where the hearing is not bad enough to justify the use of a hearing-aid, we go to a tinnitus retrainer from the outset. If we decide to try you with a hearing-aid, your first attendance ends with taking an impression of the shape of your ear canal from which an ear mould is manufactured. Alternatively, a tinnitus retrainer is ordered.'

The new patient is told that if equipment is fitted to the ear he will be seen again at regular intervals, his progress checked and a report sent to the audiological consultant who will consider whether further treatment is needed. The patient can also ask to see the consultant again. Weekly relaxation classes are on offer as are the services of a clinical psychologist for counselling. Further appointments with the clinic can be made by phone or through the post. The patients' booklet is a model of its kind in the whole of tinnitus care.

All this excellent medical attention in Nottingham is praiseworthy in itself, but it stands out as a beacon of comfort and sanity in the wasteland that comprises tinnitus management across most of the UK. If you are unfortunate enough to be seeking assistance in a typical ENT department without these standards, it is worth remembering what Nottingham provides and, perhaps with other people, asking for the local facilities to be raised to a similar level.

Find out if another hospital is better than your own, and try to be sent there. But be prepared to discover that recent and continuing reforms in NHS financing will sometimes create their own obstacles. Cost-conscious hospital trusts have so far shown no signs of giving tinnitus a higher priority when establishing budgets alongside medical needs. As it is usually a chronic condition offering little prospect of visible and recordable 'successes' it is likely to languish still deeper in the neglected areas of medicine. The chances of co-ordinated clinics springing up, even where new hospitals are opened, are not great. You can do your bit by adding your voice to local community watchdogs and pressure groups. They might even welcome the sheer novelty of adding tinnitus to their campaigns for better services, and you will find lots of neighbours—sufferers and their families—backing you.

Family doctors who now have budgets to work to may find that referral of tinnitus cases to out-patient departments is not, in their opinion, the best use of resources. They can, though, exercise greater choice in where to refer a patient (assuming they are willing to do so), so finding the better type of hospital could become easier.

## A TINNITUS MANIFESTO

Since 1992 the private sounds inside the heads of millions of people in the UK have been joined by a chorus of publicly heard voices demanding that tinnitus be taken more seriously. Sufferers have rallied behind what has been hailed as a manifesto for change, the Tinnitus Charter 2000, whose sheer novelty is likely to win it a place in the history of the struggle against tinnitus. Incredibly there had never before been a similar document setting out the extent and nature of the condition and explicitly listing what should be done for relief and cure. It seeks 'a better deal for the 4 million people in the UK who suffer persistent internal head noises, through improved medical attention to secure management of the disorder and increased medical research funding towards an ultimate cure'. The document adds: 'Generations of tinnitus sufferers have been neglected by society. The burden adults and children continue to bear is little understood by the rest of the population and the provision of public resource, for both treatment in the National Health Service and the work of researchers, is scandalously low. An aim of Tinnitus Charter 2000 is to break this debilitating circle of private ignorance and public neglect by the end of the century. To achieve this, some immediate action needs to be taken.'

The Charter, welcomed by lay and medical people, calls upon the Government, the medical and social professions, community leaders and interested members of the public to support, in intention and implementation, the following nine requests:

1  Greater funding of the Medical Research Council to extend current tinnitus research.
2  The creation of more tinnitus-only clinics throughout the UK.
3  Greater acceptance of severe tinnitus as a handicap, in granting of unemployment, disability and other welfare benefits.
4  Free and universal provision of ear-worn tinnitus maskers to sufferers capable of finding relief from them.
5  A higher priority place for tinnitus in the allocation of individual hospital budgets.
6  Training of GPs and other doctors to include greater emphasis on tinnitus management.
7  Stricter control of excessive noise, which is known to cause tinnitus, in workplaces.
8  Maximum sound levels to be placed in discotheques, to protect young people.
9  Health education programmes to warn of excessive noise, and makers and retailers of home discos and audio equipment to endorse the warning.

Charter 2000 has received wide support in both Houses of Parliament, with numerous MPs and peers pledging their active help in pursuing its aims. Trade union organisations see it as a public expression of many of their own members' dissatisfaction at the difficulties they face in receiving adequate compensation for tinnitus brought on by dangerously noisy workplaces. Ex-servicemen's organisations have used it to support their call for compensation to be paid for tinnitus arising from duties in the armed forces. It has also helped to place the subject more prominently in the media, with some national journals publishing what is believed to be their first coverage of tinnitus.

In other respects it has so far done little to dent the solid wall of ignorance, and even hostility, from which tinnitus has suffered for so long. Though it has been properly briefed in recent years, with statistics available from the Institute of Hearing Research, the Government has shown little signs of doing anything positive about tinnitus, or even understanding its magnitude. 'It is not known how many people have tinnitus,' a Health Minister told a questioner in the House of Commons in January 1995. 'The number of tinnitus-only clinics are not available centrally. However, there are facilities for the treatment of tinnitus at all the National Health Service ear, nose and throat departments. As with all patient groups, responsibility for the provision of services for people with tinnitus rests with the health authorities who have to assess needs and priorities against resources. We have no plans to review these provisions.'

The outlook for tinnitus thus remains bleak in areas where politics and medicine merge. There are no signs that ministers favour any national initiatives to help fight it. They excuse the inaction by defending the autonomy enjoyed by the area health authorities, who must locally decide if money and personnel should be diverted to treating the condition. Where national action would be appropriate there has also been a disappointing response to the campaign for a fair deal for tinnitus sufferers and for measures to prevent the spread of the condition. War veterans still find it hard to get compensation; anyone unable to work is unlikely to obtain financial help, which is more readily available to those with visible disabilities; and anti-noise laws for the workplace still do not cover places of entertainment.

Lack of sympathy is also encountered in the music and entertainment industries. Whenever the subject of pop concerts and discos and their potential to give tinnitus to young people is aired publicly, some promoters and disco owners have bluntly challenged the argument, saying there is no evidence to prove that loud sounds enjoyed by young people ever cause permanent noises in the head. Suppliers of home stereo equipment are just as unfriendly to the Tinnitus Charter, continuing to advertise the 'head blasting' and 'mind blowing' qualities of some amplifiers and loud speakers.

Campaigners have been dismayed at the widespread ignorance among people whose job it is to understand medical problems. Some doctors writing advice columns in magazines and newspapers play down the seriousness of tinnitus, describing it as 'just a ringing in the ear' and 'something that can be a bit annoying' but can be forgotten. A medical pundit on a morning TV programme attracted hundreds of letters and phone calls from viewers, mostly sufferers themselves, when he implied that it was nothing more than a temporary problem caused by the build-up of wax in the ear. Medical journalists who can write with accuracy and fluency about obscure ailments affecting a tiny number of people struggle to describe this unpleasant condition experienced to some extent by one in ten of their readers.

Neglect of tinnitus in public health provision and ignorance of it among the public at large seem to feed on each other. If people knew more about it, there would be more pressure on the NHS to do more. If the Government were to highlight it in the publicity which pours from the Department of Health, public ignorance would evaporate. Meanwhile any attention is largely eclipsed by the drama and medico-glamour of such developments as replacement surgery and pharmaceutical advances against the killer diseases. Invisible sounds which cannot be measured or understood, and which lacked a campaigning voice until the early 1990s, must form the basis of a powerful argument for public awareness and action. The ordinary person needs to know about tinnitus to appreciate what his fellow citizens have to bear. The policy- and decision-makers should know enough to begin to cure the chronic neglect of tinnitus.

There are some grounds for hope. The word TINNITUS is

now on more people's lips than before, as it creeps from the shadows. This is partly due to the burgeoning realisation that people can play a bigger role in securing and maintaining their own health. Awareness of the dangers of loud sounds, and consequently of tinnitus, is in an unexpected way riding in the wake of the layman's increased opinions about unconnected topics like dieting and skin cancer. There is a fashion for, perhaps an abiding switch to, good health, and tinnitus can benefit from this.

Should tinnitus ever become a fashionable topic enjoying greater media exposure, sufferers—including public figures—will be inclined to talk more openly about it. They can put away their shyness, shame or other causes of their reluctance to speak out and join what campaigners for a cure are now calling their crusade for silence.

One person who long ago decided to speak out is Lord Ashley of Stoke, better known as Jack Ashley MP, who has conducted justly famed campaigns on behalf of the disabled. After an unsuccessful operation to cure slight deafness he lost his hearing in the 1960s and acquired loud and permanent tinnitus. He was encouraged to stay in the House of Commons where he remained until 1992, winning world notoriety as a totally deaf member of a national legislature. He is now prominent in the Tinnitus Campaign and speaks articulately of the sheer awfulness of his noises. 'If hearts can be transplanted, why not a cure for tinnitus?' he often asks. When his sounds shattered his life Lord Ashley was thought to have a future as a government minister. He is warmly admired and respected in both Houses of Parliament and his advocacy is contributing to whittling away the indifference to tinnitus among the legislators.

It is in another law-making assembly that real progress may well be made. As the European Union goes ahead with harmonisation of so many laws, the European Parliament is being asked to recognise the nature of tinnitus and consider multi-national action in the field of health and social welfare. British MEPs have already been fully briefed on the subject and a petition will be presented to the Parliament before the next Euro elections. Increased power being given to Euro MPs partly involves health and social services. There is, therefore, a real possibility that member states of the EU will be expected in future years to deal with tinnitus on a par with other medical conditions, in the provision of treatment and social benefits. Environmental directives could also place limits on permitted decibel levels in places of public entertainment. European Union countries together have millions of citizens whose normal life is badly affected, to the point of not being able to follow the career of their choice or work at all. No one has attempted to evaluate the economic cost to the national economy of any country. When the calculations are made for Europe as a whole, the case for action on economic grounds will be overwhelming, quite apart from the humanitarian argument.

# 8   The Search for a Cure

The most remarkable feature of tinnitus research is its youth. Ancient Egyptian and Assyrian physicians knew that some people had noises in the head and offered primitive treatments. It would be good to record that progress roughly kept pace with scientific enlightenment, but it did not. Modern tinnitus research dates astonishingly from just the first half of the 1970s.

The progress that has been made in the short space of two decades can be attributed largely to the pioneering work of an American hearing specialist, Jack Vernon, and a few of his colleagues in Portland, Oregon. They, and others, are still not yet in sight of defeating tinnitus, but their continuing efforts have, more than anything, made tinnitus a serious case for investigation. Many lines of research are now being explored in several countries, but Vernon can be credited with pioneering the technique of sound-masking of tinnitus. The London researcher and surgeon Jonathan Hazell acknowledges the work as establishing 'the first attempt to do anything about tinnitus apart from telling patients to go away and "learn to live with it". Countless patients over the world owe him a debt of gratitude for the relief that masking brought them when there was nothing else.' He describes his American colleague, with whom he works closely, as a 'trail blazer at a time when it was considered professional suicide to engage in tinnitus research'.

Some doctors think the less said about the subject the better, as talking about its horrors only makes it worse for serious sufferers. Vernon has no such reticence, and his statement that 'nothing robs Man of the quality of life in the manner which tinnitus does' has been repeated often by those campaigning for wider recognition of it. Lord Ashley, with decades of bad tinnitus behind him, must surely have had Vernon in mind when he once said that 'only those affected and a handful of experts appreciate the intensity of tinnitus suffering'. Outside the widening circle of international research, Vernon has also won a huge lay audience among America's estimated 50 million people suffering from tinnitus, in the advice he gives them in the pages of *Tinnitus Today*, the journal of the American Tinnitus Association.

Twenty years is not long, of course, in medical research, especially in view of the baffling difficulties and mysteries of an affliction such as tinnitus. Researchers today must be seen realistically as pioneers. It may be that only future generations of sufferers will enjoy the fruits of present studies. The slowness of progress cannot be blamed solely on the sheer scientific complexities facing the few who research tinnitus; lack of financial support from official quarters has remained an obstacle, nowhere more so than in Britain. Governments and their advisers have repeatedly declined to regard tinnitus as a separate subject with a claim on public funds. To its disadvantage, the problem of head sounds has been subordinated and obscured by the subject of deafness, in such areas as hospital treatment and payment of military pensions. In research, it suffers in the same manner.

Around £3 million of taxpayers' money goes each year to the Institute of Hearing Research, via the Medical Research Council. No other money is paid by the Government specifically for tinnitus work, and the Institute is at liberty to decide how much, or how little, should be devoted to tinnitus. While it has been argued that research aimed at curing deafness could be of some benefit to tinnitus, the Institute has only allocated some £120,000 a year to tinnitus research—or less than 3p for every adult and child waiting for a cure in the UK. In 1993, moreover, work on tinnitus at the Institute was reduced, in its own words, to 'a pilot light' following staff changes—a decision supported by the Government. In the realm of public funding, then, the research diet in the immediate future looks like continuing to be small crumbs from the rich table.

Tinnitus projects outside the Institute of Hearing Research have a battle to survive. Although their costs are generally modest, they often keep going from year to year by seeking help from charitable foundations and industry.

With tinnitus research but a couple of decades old, it is too early to say in what broader area a breakthrough is likely to be made. To date the programmes of desensitising and retraining the brain being worked on by Jonathan Hazell's team in London, and elsewhere, offer the most promise, not least because this therapy is the only treatment yet to claim total remission, albeit in a small number of cases. Its weakness seems to be in the required commitment and co-operation of the patients themselves, and in the lack of sufficient trained people able to give the therapy.

Anyone with loud enough noises may well promise to cooperate in a treatment programme suggested by doctors and therapists, but this often demands an active and persistent role well beyond the strength and staying power of many. And there are problems in imparting advice to tinnitus sufferers who are profoundly deaf, or simultaneously battling with psychological or psychiatric problems unconnected with their tinnitus. Anything that makes face-to-face communication between patient and therapist difficult, such as language differences, is bound to challenge retraining the brain as a universal form of relief. It should be encouraged, but unfortunately should be regarded as nothing more than a narrow and restricted path to silence.

Surgery has little to offer. Very rarely it is found that tinnitus is brought about by a disorder in the middle ear or by something wrong with the blood vessels or muscles inside or close to the ear. In such cases an operation has been known to eliminate the head sounds completely. In the more

complex inner ear, however, the surgeon is unable to intervene in the malfunction of hair cells and nerves.

Trail-blazing work being led by a young researcher in
the laboratories of Keele University is attracting universal
attention and could be of unprecedented benefit for people
with tinnitus or deafness. Its main purpose is to stimulate
the growth of damaged hair cells in the inner ear. Damage to
the cells in the highly sensitive cochlea, or to their nerve
connections to the brain, is believed to be the cause of some
tinnitus, as well as deafness in millions of people. The
auditory neuro-anatomy group at Keele, led by Dr Carole
Hackney, is hoping to provide greater understanding of how
the inner ear works and exactly what happens when it is
damaged. Using powerful electron microscopes, one magnifying the ear 100,000 times, the scientists are exploring
three main areas. First, they are investigating how the hair
cells can turn the vibrations from sound in the cochlea into
the vital nerve signals sent to the brain. 'Understanding this
mechanism and how its sensitivity is determined could help
us find out whether hair cells ever send inappropriate
messages to the brain, which is one possible cause of
tinnitus,' says Dr Hackney. 'Secondly, we are investigating which neurotransmitter chemicals the nerve cells in
the auditory pathway use to send signals to each other.
It has been suggested that over-release of an excitatory
neurotransmitter, glutamate, could be one cause of tinnitus.'
The researchers are finding that it is this neurotransmitter
that is used by the auditory nerve to transmit information to
the brain. 'This is important because drugs being developed
in other laboratories to safely block nerve signals mediated
by glutamate in other parts of the brain may turn out to be
useful in treating tinnitus or hyperacusis [over-sensitivity to
sound],' Dr Hackney explains.

The third area of research at Keele concerns recovery
from hearing loss. Certain strong antibiotics have been
known for some time to cause damage to hair cells and
thus bring about deafness. Mechanical disturbances to the

cochlea could well lead to tinnitus. Deafness brought about by the antibiotics has usually been regarded as permanent, but it has recently been shown that guinea pigs deafened in this way can show partial or complete recovery of their hearing. The regrowth of damaged hair cells could one day return a disordered human ear to normality and banish some forms of tinnitus.

The belief that one day medicines will provide some, or most, tinnitus cures lies behind important research being done at Birmingham University. A homeopathic medicine called 'Tinnitus' is being investigated as part of a variety of work on the pharmaceutical treatment of head noises. Its ingredients are those which some people associate with the cause or aggravation of tinnitus. In the first controlled trials of the medicine, volunteers had to avoid coffee, tea and anything which contained caffeine. Some reduction in tinnitus was recorded among a number of people.

Patients recovering consciousness after operations unconnected with tinnitus have sometimes found that their head sounds have disappeared, but return again after a short while. This has prompted experiments, and researchers have been encouraged to find that the anaesthetic lignocaine, when given in small doses by injection into a vein, will temporarily abolish or reduce tinnitus. It is not yet a viable ongoing treatment, but the search is on for a parallel drug which can both be taken by mouth and is capable of giving more than transient relief. It is not known exactly how lignocaine can bring silence, however temporarily. Conversely, and in rare cases, a general anaesthetic is believed to have caused or worsened tinnitus.

The recent advances in the study of neuro-anatomy could be highly important. Greater understanding of the nature and function of nerves will be followed by more drugs, some of which will one day probably enable highly selective correction of inner ear nerves and perception of sounds by the brain. The first step could be the voluntary deafening of a patient with the simultaneous abolition of the tinnitus, and from that it is not fanciful to envisage a narrowing of the target to check the tinnitus only.

Researchers throughout the world increasingly exchange their latest theories and findings, and every four years an international seminar is held for scientific investigators and practitioners.

The sheer variety of the work being conducted from country to country is reassuring, but perhaps also serves to show how little agreement there is on which form of research holds most promise. It also strengthens the belief that tinnitus, as a symptom of a number of underlying disorders, requires not one but several cures.

A German doctor runs a deliberately luxurious residential clinic where comfort is seen as a vital factor. While patients are enjoying food and surroundings to match the most expensive of hotels, they undergo psychotherapy and other treatments. Some of the most distressed patients respond well and quickly, finding themselves better equipped to handle their tinnitus and reporting some reduction of it. The multi-disciplinary approach in luxurious surroundings is extremely costly, but is being taken seriously as a line of treatment with possibilities. Also in Germany, sufferers who find it difficult to sleep have been fitted with hearing-aids connected with wires through which natural sounds and music are fed.

At the Welsh Institute of Hearing Research in Cardiff, a number of suicides, which may have been caused by tinnitus reaching an intolerable level, have been studied. It has been found that depression plays a vital role in the decision of anyone to contemplate suicide. Taking one's own life remains extremely uncommon among sufferers who do not already have significant psychiatric disturbance.

American researchers have reported partial success in the use of the tranquilliser alprazolam (trade name Xanax), with a number of patients finding some benefit. In the opinion of some tinnitus specialists in the UK the feeling of relief could probably be achieved by almost any tranquillisers.

They also warn that such drugs can be easily addictive.

In Sweden, work continues on establishing links between jaw disorders and tinnitus, but without conclusive results.

French scientists are looking at the control the brain exerts on the function of the inner ear via the nerve pathways. Deeper knowledge in this field is expected to lead to greater understanding of tinnitus generation.

In Israel, some evidence has emerged of a deficiency of vitamin B12 in military personnel with bad noise-induced tinnitus. The same team of researchers have found that self-hypnosis can help some sufferers.

Epidemiological studies are made in various countries. In Singapore it has been found that 23 per cent of people with noise-induced deafness also have tinnitus. The same people tended to have rather worse hearing than those without tinnitus, confirming observations made earlier in Canada and the UK.

The danger of exposure to loud noise was studied among a number of army personnel in Finland. Half of them had less than normal hearing for their age and a third of the total had tinnitus, most of them continuously. Although the use of hearing protectors had increased in recent years, the researchers reported a large number of younger men were still suffering disabling tinnitus and deafness.

Tinnitus in animals is being investigated in the University of Maryland, USA. Rats have been given different doses of aspirin-like salicylate drugs and their responses and behaviour studied alongside other rats. Professor Pawel Jastreboff says that 'a cure remains elusive and the mechanisms of origins speculative. The crucial obstacle in tinnitus research has been the lack of an animal model'.

# 9   Tinnitus and the Future

With the brazen nerve of the most unwelcome of guests who has been shown the door but still declines to leave, tinnitus will doubtlessly crash and scream its way into a part of the twenty-first century. Just how long it will be before it is banished and walks away in shame at the havoc it has caused no one can tell. It remains as much a matter of speculation and hope among doctors and researchers as it is among a large number of suffering humanity. There is comfort in both reflecting what has been achieved and considering some of the changes and innovations needed to make a cure or cures attainable in the coming years.

Sufferers impatient for progress forgivably list the achievements of science and technology in other fields and wonder why there has been nothing for them. Older people can recall the splitting of the atom, while middle-aged people remember the first heart transplant and space walks. All had, to some extent, been derided as fanciful by experts a few years earlier. Will there not be a corresponding breakthrough for tinnitus, which will disappear or greatly diminish in a few years of dazzling activity in the laboratory and centres of health care?

The inventors and discoverers whose labours produce life-enhancing bonuses for the human race invariably are driven on by the demand for a broad or specific improvement in our lives and people articulating the need for it. This social momentum can be enough to focus resources and intellectual power which in turn produces the desired breakthrough. At first glance there is no such virtuous circle, nor the likelihood of one, working in favour of tinnitus.

It will take a social historian with a good grounding in collective psychology to explain why this ghastly scourge has escaped public opprobrium until very recent years. It is true that many people in other times remained silent in case the mention of it suggested mental derangement requiring a spell in an asylum. But that cannot be the whole story. The reason must largely lie in the nature of the affliction itself. Tinnitus involves the highly subjective sense of hearing, and it cannot be shared. Explaining it to the world at large is therefore just as difficult now as it has ever been. Any description of it to a non-sufferer is doomed by its own inadequacy; there is as yet no real medium of communication to convey the message to the most sympathetic listener willing to learn. A tape of simulated sounds of tinnitus now goes a long way towards bridging the gap of incomprehension in a manner denied to earlier generations. Conveying what it is like to have to live with it remains an impossible task, as it is essentially an inner annoyance or anxiety, with the sounds being nothing more than the perceived cause. In brief, there is no language or method of communication quite up to the task. Persuasive prose, stirring poetry, anguished painting and drawing have all been enlisted by sufferers through the generations to tell the rest of the world about it. Their efforts serve often as therapy of self-expression, but not much else. Tinnitus, through those who bear it, does dare to speak its name, but cannot fully do so. It has not yet found the right words.

For as long as tinnitus stays an unexpressed problem, beyond the factual definitions of dictionaries and the inadequate words of individuals, progress towards its solution will remain frustratingly slow. So society must not only be told about it, but taught how to regard it, short of actual experience. How this can be done is best learned by comparing public attitudes to other medical conditions. Commonly the catalyst of sympathy and understanding is physical pain. Knowledge of another person's painful illness can be heightened by recollections of one's own trivial anguish caused by perhaps a hammer blow to a finger. The pain and trauma of another's severe accident can be imagined alongside one's own memories of a cut caused by a broken glass in the kitchen or a slight burn from a saucepan. There is a gulf between the experiences in seriousness and severity, but there is a common language of pain.

People groping for the right expression to do justice to their head sounds sometimes talk of the 'sound of pain' or the 'pain of sound'. Should anyone think the words are an exaggeration, they should know that noise above 140 decibels is actually felt as pain by anyone close to it without protection for their ears. As far as it can be measured at all, tinnitus is reckoned to be well below that level, but the subjective hearing of it day and night brings an infinitely greater discomfort than a slight physical 'painful' accident. Pain, therefore, can legitimately be used as a deserving description of tinnitus, and not just as an analogy or metaphor. The general public then may at last accept it for what it is—a painful affliction deserving attention and the resources to defeat it.

If, overnight, the public were to be aware of the awfulness and extent of tinnitus, one would hope that there would be an eruption of wrath at its academic and scientific neglect. Would, for instance, the absence of a well-equipped national centre of research be quietly accepted? Why is there no single establishment where the quest for a relief and ultimate cure can be housed and co-ordinated? There would certainly be surprise to find that the setting up of such an establishment would be viewed with less than delight by some people already engaged in tinnitus research. As in many branches of research, there is a preference for separated studies at some hospitals and universities. Personal ambitions and professional pride are not always subservient to the greater cause of the alleviation of suffering. Pooling of resources and ideas does not always commend itself to researchers who understandably and quietly defend their own distinct areas of study.

The creation of a national institute of tinnitus research (perhaps, one day, that will be its title) would require nothing less than a sea change in the traditional system of centrally-directed medical research in the UK. The Government finances its Medical Research Council, which in turn allocates funds to research projects. It appears to be an orderly way of managing things, except that governments are thus able to shed responsibility for the neglect of something like tinnitus research by saying that the Council must make the final decisions. While the role of government over many decades has become increasingly interventionist in directing the economic and social life of the nation, it has chosen to adopt a more than arm's-length approach to fundamental research capable of bettering the lives of millions of its citizens. There never will be a case for politicians to control branches of science which require the researcher to have the freedom to proceed along the most promising path. There is, however, an argument for them to decide which areas of medical research require attention and to what extent money and facilities should be made available. Until popular pressure builds up to an irresistible force, and Parliament feels it is time to intervene and indicate whether a particular medical affliction deserves a bigger part of the nation's wealth, tinnitus will suffer neglect. Governments do legislate and ministers do use their permanent executive powers to influence many aspects of public health. When it comes to fundamental aspects of medical research, however, they are happy to remain impotent and unwilling to identify and act upon major medical problems.

The arm's-length attitude of our elected representatives is equally visible and deplorable in the running of the National Health Service. The Exchequer provides billions of pounds to the NHS, but is unwilling to lay down guidelines for treatment of a particular ailment or handicap. With a minister unblushingly telling the House of Commons that there is not even a central Whitehall record of the number of tinnitus clinics operating in public hospitals, let alone where they can be found, it means that the Government cannot do more than guess what is on offer for sufferers.

It is hard to see how the situation can be improved with greater autonomy and financial accountability being handed to hospital trusts in the NHS. Patients, none the less, are being urged to look upon themselves as customers, rather than passive recipients of whatever treatment is on hand. Consumerism is edging its way into the NHS, and in the coming years tinnitus people—as much as any other group of patients—will have a louder voice in demanding a better deal in ear, nose and throat departments and, eventually, in separate tinnitus clinics. Referrals to hospital clinics will continue to be made mainly by family doctors, whose medical training now hardly includes any reference to tinnitus or knowledge of how to handle it in the surgery. As the public's awareness rises there will be pressure to give it more attention in the medical curriculum. When this happens there will be a corresponding interest in audiology as an area of specialism, and with it greater attention paid to tinnitus. At the moment there is little inducement for new doctors to choose tinnitus as a lifetime subject for treatment or research, as it lacks glamour, finance and prestige. Its long-awaited transformation will be said to have happened when head noises are elevated to serious academic status, the world's first professorial chair is devoted to their study and the word 'tinnitology' enters the lexicon of medicine.

There is no corner so dark that it will escape for ever the light of Mankind's expanding knowledge; tinnitus will give up its dark secrets. There is no horror so profound that it will defy for ever the undying spirit of human struggle against the sternest of enemies; tinnitus will yield.

The coming decades offer hope for us, where previous generations of sufferers lived and died in ignorance and solitary despair. The world's millions suffering with head sounds today have a hitherto unequalled opportunity to seek and find relief. They should also resolve to demand, for themselves and for future sufferers, living and as yet unborn, a larger share of the medical and scientific wealth of the world to relieve and conquer their affliction. Their voices will turn the crying anguish of the past and present into a chorus of hope for a future of blissful silence.

# The British Tinnitus Association

It is a historical truth of which we can boast that Britain has led the world in what may be called 'formal charity'. Thanks to the tradition of Victorian philanthropy—however condescending that was to the deserving masses—good causes have flourished since the nineteenth century. Foreigners will often remark that, compared with their own countries, the UK seems to have a well-intentioned association for almost everything, ready to rattle a collection box on a flag day or touch the public conscience in some other way.

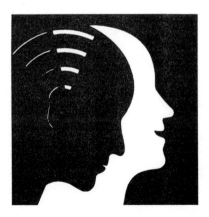

Those dedicated to the relief and cure of medical conditions are among the institutes, trusts, societies and the like jostling for public attention, sympathy and funds. Today there are some 170,000 registered charities. The smallest are of the most specialised nature affecting only a tiny section of society. The largest have multi-million budgets and all the trappings of a commercial organisation. When the big moment came for tinnitus, therefore, and its sufferers decided to speak up for themselves, they found a crowded marketplace in which to pitch their stall and sell the subject. The clamour for attention among other medical charities has been, from the start, a daunting experience. One huge problem for us has been the fact that the very name *tinnitus* is unknown to a large section of the population. Even some people with tinnitus have spent their lives totally ignorant of the word.

The public, organised battle for the relief and cure of head noises can be dated from July 1979 when a meeting in a committee room of the House of Commons decided an organisation should be set up. The man behind it was a Labour backbench MP, Jack (now Lord) Ashley, himself a tinnitus sufferer and campaigner extraordinary on behalf of the disabled. His constant head sounds and deafness had all but finished his parliamentary career in the previous decade. Countless people with similar or other disabilities have found his unbroken success in public life an unmatched inspiration to fight back against the odds. His work for tinnitus has certainly helped to pull many from the precipice of despair and surrender.

His inaugural meeting of The British Tinnitus Association (BTA) was important and significant enough to earn it a footnote in the history of twentieth-century medical and charitable endeavour. It was plainly a life-enhancing event for people who had put up with their ghastly burden over the years and now heard that a national body was in existence devoted wholly to their well-being. 'For the first time in my life I cried with joy,' said a seventy-eight-year-old woman in Scotland. 'The sun shone for me when I read that something was being done.' Someone else explained his feelings: 'My daughter has suffered badly for thirty years, since her childhood. The feeling of helplessness in not being able to help her has been the worst thing I have had to bear in life.'

From the start the BTA has not been in the least afraid to criticise the chronic neglect of tinnitus in the National Health Service and government-funded research. It has been unfettered by encrusted deference towards established authority which has held some older charities back from certain aspects of campaigning. All too often organisations have used their charitable status—quite unnecessarily as it has turned out—as an excuse for not pursuing a particular activity at odds with established practices or policies. An organisation, for instance, receiving an annual grant from a government department has sometimes hesitated before adopting what could be seen as a political stance more in line with that of an opposition party at Westminster. Similarly, there has been reluctance to argue with institutions outside government and Parliament, for fear of disrupting the status quo.

What has been done in an organised and campaigning fashion for tinnitus has roughly coincided with the new wave of charitable work, now generally called the Third Sector, in the larger fields of public and private enterprise. Quite a lot has happened in a few years.

In quantity the work of the BTA compares modestly with that of the major charities, but almost everything it does breaks new ground for tinnitus sufferers and finds a ready response from those who are either sufferers or who are anxious to assist in lightening the burden carried by too many for so long.

Responsibility for running the new association in 1979 was taken on by the Royal National Institute for Deaf People, which had already begun to assist the small amount of tinnitus research being undertaken. Self-help groups were set up in many towns and members were quickly recruited from people naturally hoping for a cure or instant relief. But disappointment often followed when expectations were not met. There were, in addition, basic problems in having the

RNID, whose speciality was deafness, running an organisation dealing with tinnitus. The two conditions, it is true,
occur together in some people, but many have tinnitus with
unimpaired hearing. Clearly the baffling medical condition
which was newly struggling to win a proper public airing
needed an organisation to itself. The status of poor relation
just would not do for a body potentially representing the
wishes of a tenth of the adult population.

The break came in 1991, when the BTA's branches and
individual members voted overwhelmingly to become a
totally independent charity. Membership then stood at 4,000
and it was accurately felt that growth would accelerate as
the association won its freedom to develop in its own more
purposeful way. As a new body the BTA (it kept its name) at
least had the distinct advantage of being unfettered by
tradition and was ready to take its place in—to some extent
lead—the fast-developing style of charity campaigning.

One of the first steps taken was to introduce the subject in
the House of Commons. There was an immediate and
favourable response to a briefing sent to all MPs, some of
whom admitted to having battled with tinnitus themselves
for years. Others said their wives or husbands were sufferers. A House of Commons motion was tabled, welcoming
the fact that tinnitus now had its own voice for the first time,
in the form of an exclusive campaigning charity. It was
signed by MPs from all parties.

In 1992 even more significant progress was made. The
BTA launched its Tinnitus Charter 2000 calling for better
NHS treatment, more generous funding for research and
state recognition of head noises as a disability when sufferers apply for Social Security help. It also sought to
prevent the spread of tinnitus, in part by calling for lower
sound levels in discotheques and better public education to
explain the dangers of loud noises.

The Charter, which was the first document of its kind ever
to be published on the subject was keenly received. Among
the thousands of enquiries received by the BTA was a letter

from a Somerset man who had been a serious sufferer for over half a century. 'This is the first time I have seen any publicity about what I have had to put up with since boyhood. What has the medical world been doing all this time?'

At last, the BTA told itself, tinnitus has a voice.

# The Tinnitus Population of the UK

Nearly five million adults and children in the UK have permanent head noises. Most of them are only slightly or not at all worried by it, but hundreds of thousands are so badly affected they cannot lead a normal life and many are unable to earn a living. The following table refers to men and women of seventeen and above:

|  | England | N. Ireland | Scotland | Wales |
|---|---|---|---|---|
| Total with tinnitus | 3,800,000 | 120,000 | 400,000 | 230,000 |
| Moderately annoyed | 950,000 | 30,000 | 100,000 | 57,500 |
| Quality of life severely affected | 380,000 | 12,000 | 40,000 | 23,000 |
| Normal life severely affected | 190,000 | 6,000 | 20.000 | 11,500 |

Statistics based on the UK National Study of Hearing, researched over several years and including a household study in 1982–3.

# Useful Addresses

## General information and advice

The British Tinnitus Association
14–18 West Bar Green, Sheffield, SA1 2DA.
Tel: 01142 796600

Hearing Research Trust
530 Gray's Inn Road, London WC1X 8EE.
Tel: 0171 833 1733

Royal National Institute for Deaf People
105, Gower Street, London WC1E 6AH.
Tel: 0171 387 8033

## Information on tinnitus hazards in the workplace

Health and Safety Executive
Secretariat:
Baynards House, Chepstow Place, London W2 4TF.
Tel: 0171 243 6000

Also:
Stanley Precinct, Bootle, Merseyside.
Tel: 0151 951 4000

## Suppliers of tinnitus maskers and/or hearing-aids

Sarabec Ltd
15 High Force Road, Middlesbrough, Cleveland TS2 1RH.
Tel: 01642 247789
(Also video subtitling and other domestic equipment)

Bonochord Hearing Aids
5 Sevenoaks Business Centre, Cramptons Road,
Sevenoaks, Kent TN14 5DQ.
Tel: 01732 457668

Starkey Laboratories Ltd
Meridian House, Bramhall Technology Park, Pepper Road,
Hazel Grove, Stockport, Cheshire SK7 5BX.
Tel: 0161 483 2200

Williams Tinnitus Maskers
67a Bexley High Street, Bexley, Kent DA5 1AA.
Tel: 01322 558596

AudiMed
Enterprise House, 511–513 Upper Elmers End Road,
Beckenham, Kent BR3 3DB.
Tel: 0181 663 0760

DM Marketing
PO Box 1200, Benfleet, Essex SS7 1JY.
Tel: 01268 565888

Cubex
25 New Cavendish Street, London W1M 8LP
Tel: 0171 935 5511

**Therapeutic Treatments**

Chartered Society of Physiotherapy
14 Bedford Square, London WC1R 4ED.
Tel: 0171 242 1941

British Society of Medical and Dental Hypnosis
42 Links Road, Ashtead, Surrey.
Tel: 01372 273522

Tomatis Centre UK
3 Wallands Crescent, Lewes, East Sussex BN7 2QT.
Tel: 01273 474877

Cranio-sacral Therapy Association
Stillpoint, Whiteways, Stroud, Gloucestershire GL6 7EP.
Tel: 01285 821648

The Craniofacial Pain Clinic
42 Harley Street, London W1.
Tel: 0171 637 5797

The Shiatsu Society
5 Foxcote, Wokingham, Berkshire RG11 3PG.
Tel: 01734 730 836

Osteopathic Information Service
PO Box 2074, Reading, Berkshire RG1 4YR.
Tel: 01734 512051

British Chiropractic Association
29 Whitley Street, Reading, Berkshire RG2 0EG.
Tel: 01734 757557

Register of Traditional Chinese Medicine
19 Trinity Road, London N2 8JJ.
Tel: 0181 883 8431

## Tinnitus-based pensions for ex-servicemen and women

War Pensions Branch
DSS, B North Fylde Central Office,
Norcross, Blackpool FY5 3TA.

War Pensions Office (Northern Ireland)
Marlborough House, 30 Victoria Street, Belfast BT1 3GE.

Ministry of Defence F2 (Air)
Building 56, RAF Innsworth, Gloucester GL3 1HW.

Royal Navy and Royal Marines
Ministry of Defence NPP (Accounts), 3A, HMS Centurian,
Grange Road, Gosport PO13 9XA.

# Index

acupressure 76–7
acupuncture 73–6
adult education courses 25
age factors 11–12
alarm-clocks 40
alcohol 89, 90–1
alprazolam 133
alternative therapies 68–80
American Tinnitus Association 129
anaesthetics, general 132
antibiotics 59, 131, 132
anti-fungal drugs 57
anxiety 85, 90, 95, 96
arthritis 56, 60
artistic expression 25–6
Ashley, Lord 126, 127, 129, 142
aspirin 98
attitudes to tinnitus 99–101
auditory subcortex 19
automatic gain control (AGC)
    46–7

Beethoven, L. von 7–8, 60
benefits 112–14
Benefits Agency 113
benzodiazepine 56
bereavement 61
Birmingham and District Tinnitus
    Group 34
Birmingham University 132
blood pressure 58
brain 26, 78
British Association for Counselling
    52

British Psychological Association
    52
British Tinnitus Association 19,
    84, 103, 141–5
Building Research Establishment
    63

Callas, M. 71
Cambridge University 45–6
cannabis 61
captioning for television 42
cassette players 41
CD player 41
chiropractic 65–6
cholesterol 58
cochlea 3, 98, 131, 132
compensation, claiming 110–12
complementary medicine 83;
    see also names of specific
    types
counselling 51–3
craniofacial therapy 79–80
cranio-sacral massage 77–9
cure, search for 128–34
cycling 25

deafening, voluntary 132–3
deafness 28, 29, 36, 73, 94
    disability 116–17
    noise-induced 134
    total 28–32, 130
decibel levels 14–15, 107, 108,
    109–10
deep heat therapy 56

dental fillings   58–9
dentistry   58–9
Depardieu, G.   71
Department of Education   16
Department of Health   125
Department of Social Security
     117
depression   5, 65
diazepam   56
diet   89–91
   high-fat   89
disco music   13–15, 62
distress   81
Dixon, D.   9
dizziness   56
doctors' reactions to tinnitus   18,
     23, 26, 50–1
door signals   38
drugs   56, 57, 61, 64, 65, 67, 131,
     133, 134
   treatment   98

ear:
   brain link   5, 12
   care   91–3
   drops   92
   drum   4, 102
   hypersensitive   94–6
   inner   4, 19, 29, 56, 60, 61, 78,
        93, 95, 131
   middle   3, 4, 60, 71, 98, 102,
        130
   protectors   109, 110
earphones   39
education about tinnitus   14, 16
education problems because of
     17
electrical treatment   64–5
electricity   98
electro-magnetic fields   98
Electronic Ear   72
emotional strain   61, 85
environment   97–8
Eustachian tubes, obstruction of
     62, 102, 103

exasperation   104
exhaustion   104
'Executive Ear'   72

family   104
   help for   33
   reactions   29
   suggestions for   34–6
   support   32–7
fluoridisation   60
flying   33, 101–4
folk remedies   62–3

gadgets   38–49, 95
   for the home   38–42
*Gingko biloba*   57–8
glaucoma   54, 55
glucose-laced drinks   86
glutamate   131
Gogh, V. van   7
Goya, F. de   7
grommets   62

habituating to tinnitus   26–7
Hackney, C.   131
Hardy, T.   7
Hazell, J.   18, 19, 20, 21, 22, 128,
     130
head injuries   61
headphones   41
Health and Safety Executive
     108
hearing   20–1, 54, 57
   hearing-aids   39, 40, 42–7, 48,
        61, 64, 80, 97, 102, 121, 133
   tests   109
Hearing Research Trust   47
herbal medicine   62
heredity   16–17
Hewitson, E.   34
high-pressure pumping   98
Hitler, A.   6
hums   63–4
hyperacusis   94–5
hypnotism   68–71

ignorance 125
incapacity benefit 112–14
infections 57, 61
influenza 61
infra-red systems 38
insomnia 5, 41, 65
Institute of Hearing Research 124, 129, 130

jaw disorders 60, 79, 80, 134

Keele University 131

legal issues 107–17
lignocaine 132
lip reading 36, 37
loop systems 40
low energy treatment 56
LSD 61
Luxon, B. 9

Maclennan, R. 9
magnetic resonance imaging 57
Maryland, University of 134
maskers 47–9, 80, 95, 97, 102
    suppliers 148
massage 82
McKenna, L. 53
mechanical aids 38–49
Medical Research Council 123, 129, 138
meditation 82
Ménière's disease 67
Middlesex Hospital 19
migraine 54, 55
music 83–4

National Captioning Institute 42
National Health Service 48, 49, 58, 118, 119, 120, 121, 122, 125
neck disorders 55, 60, 63
nervous breakdowns 64–5
neurotransmitter chemicals 131
Noise at Work Regulations 108
noise control equipment 109

noise, loud 11, 13, 14, 28, 126, 134
noisy environment 59–60
Nottingham Tinnitus Clinic 35, 36, 120
Nottingham University NHS Hospital 120, 121

osteopathy 55–6, 60, 65, 66, 78, 80
otosclerosis 60–1
outdoor activities 23–4
outside activities 35, 105

pensions 112, 116–17, 150
physiotherapy 56, 60, 63, 77
pillow vibrators 40
politics 124
prostate disorders 64
psychological conditioning and treatment 21–2, 27–8, 87–8, 101, 133
public attitude to 29–31
public health provision 118–22, 125–6

*Quiet* 19

radar 98
radios 38, 39, 41, 49, 55
reading-lamp 41
Reagan, R. 9
reassurance 34
reflexology 65
relaxation, importance of 27, 79, 80, 81, 82–5, 97, 105, 121
relief 18–37
rheumatism 54
road accidents 63
Royal Ear Hospital 19
Royal National Institute for Deaf People 143
running 24–5
Rushdie, S. 7

Schumann, R. 8
self-help 22–6

Shiatsu 76–7
silence, total 43
sinusitis 61
sleep 88–90, 105
  inducement 41, 49
Smetana, B. 8
social issues 107–27
sodium fluoride 61
sound hallucination 96–9
spontaneous otoacoustic emissions
    (SOAEs) 98
Streisand, B. 9
stress 20, 27, 65, 71, 72, 78, 80,
    81, 82, 83, 84, 90, 95
suction machines 93
suicides 133
sugary drinks 86
surgery 3, 19, 30, 130
syringing 61, 92–3

tapes, tinnitus-masking 41
teenagers 55; *see also* disco music
telephones 40, 64
television 38, 39, 41, 42
temperomandibular disorder
    (TMJ) 79–80
temporal bone tightness 78
tension 27, 56, 77, 78
  physical 82
Therapak 41–2
therapeutic noise 48–9
therapeutic treatments 149
therapeutic wideband noise
    (WBN) 20–1
'Tinnitus' (drug) 132
tinnitus:
  definition 1
  generators 21

history of 6
Manifesto 122–7
musical 96–9
objective 98
onset 10–12, 16–17
peaks and troughs 85–8
prevalency 5–6, 146
search for cure 128–34
symptoms 108
Tinnitus Charter 2000 122, 123,
    124, 125, 144
*Tinnitus Today* 129
Tomatis, A. 71
Tomatis Method 71–3
tranquillisers 133
transcutaneous electrical neural
    stimulations (TENS) 80
transient periods of relief 23

Vernon, J. 128, 129
vitamin B12 134

waking 86, 87
walking 106
Walkmans 13
war pensions 116, 150
war wounds, tinnitus as 114–17
wax in ears 92, 93
Welsh Institute of Hearing Research
    133
whiplash injuries 63
white noise generator 96, 97
wine 28

Xanax 133
X-ray 106

young people 12–17, 62